FAST FACTS ABOUT PRESSURE ULCER CARE FOR NURSES

How to Prevent, Detect, and Resolve Them in a Nutshell

Mary Ellen Dziedzic, MSN, RN, CWOCN

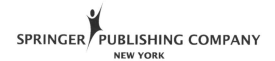

SPRINGER PUBLISHING COMPANY
NEW YORK

Springer Publishing Company, LLC
11 West 42nd Street
New York, NY 10036
www.springerpub.com

Acquisitions Editor: Margaret Zuccarini
Composition: S4Carlisle Publishing Services

ISBN: 978-0-8261-9894-5
e-book ISBN: 978-0-8261-9895-2

13 14 15 16 17 / 5 4 3 2 1

The author and the publisher of this Work have made every effort to use sources believed to be reliable to provide information that is accurate and compatible with the standards generally accepted at the time of publication. Because medical science is continually advancing, our knowledge base continues to expand. Therefore, as new information becomes available, changes in procedures become necessary. We recommend that the reader always consult current research and specific institutional policies before performing any clinical procedure. The author and publisher shall not be liable for any special, consequential, or exemplary damages resulting, in whole or in part, from the readers' use of, or reliance on, the information contained in this book. The publisher has no responsibility for the persistence or accuracy of URLs for external or third-party Internet websites referred to in this publication and does not guarantee that any content on such websites is, or will remain, accurate or appropriate.

Library of Congress Cataloging-in-Publication Data
Dziedzic, Mary Ellen, author.
Fast facts about pressure ulcer care for nurses : how to prevent, detect, and resolve them in a nutshell / Mary Ellen Dziedzic.
    p. ; cm.—(Fast facts)
Includes bibliographical references and index.
ISBN-13: 978-0-8261-9894-5 — ISBN-10: 0-8261-9894-5 — ISBN-13: 978-0-8261-9895-2 (e-book)
I. Title. II. Series: Fast facts.
[DNLM: 1. Pressure Ulcer—prevention & control. 2. Pressure Ulcer—nursing. 3. Pressure Ulcer—therapy. WR 598]
RL675
616.5'45—dc23   2013036135

Special discounts on bulk quantities of our books are available to corporations, professional associations, pharmaceutical companies, health care organizations, and other qualifying groups. If you are interested in a custom book, including chapters from more than one of our titles, we can provide that service as well.

For details, please contact:
Special Sales Department, Springer Publishing Company, LLC
11 West 42nd Street, 15th Floor, New York, NY 10036-8002
Phone: 877-687-7476 or 212-431-4370; Fax: 212-941-7842
E-mail: sales@springerpub.com

Printed in the United States of America by McNaughton & Gunn.

This book is dedicated to my loving family—my husband Mark and son Thaddeus. All things are possible with you. To my best four-legged friend Henry, thanks for sitting by my side as I wrote this book.

Contents

Part IV: Establishing the Environment of Skin Care Safety

Preface

Throughout my 28 years as a nurse I have had many different roles, including labor and delivery nurse, cardiac nurse, manager, educator, and eventually a wound care nurse. All the patients I cared for had the potential for skin issues and developing pressure ulcers. I did not realize how serious the issue was until I cared for a young man who seemed relatively healthy but had had surgery. This patient, though large, appeared as if he could move himself and shift his weight. Normally people will shift positions if they are in one position for a long time. Think about how many times you shift your weight when on a long trip in a car.

The patient was not moved by the nurses caring for him nor was he encouraged to move. He was walked per postoperative instructions but when he was in bed or in the chair, he essentially stayed in one position because it was too painful to move. The patient developed a very large pressure ulcer to his buttocks. The wound measured 15 cm by 15 cm. The ulcer initially started as a large purple area but eventually started to slough and became covered with thick black tissue. Once the ulcer was noted, treatment and further prevention were initiated but the ulcer was bone deep. Because the man was young, no one wanted to disturb him or offensively look at his buttocks. This young man had to have several additional surgeries to clean the wound and plastic surgery to close the wound after several months, and he had to go to a short-term rehabilitation facility as his mobility was further impeded.

This ulcer was an eye-opener—it was large and odorous, and caused the patient additional pain and discomfort, all of which could have been avoided if simple steps had been taken. It is possible to decrease facility-acquired pressure ulcers and develop an environment of safety when it comes to skin care. Through a concerted effort by all levels of employees at Geisinger Health System where I am a CWOCN and coordinator of the wound ostomy program, pressure ulcers have decreased by more than 75% with the incidence of Stage III and Stage IV ulcers decreasing to zero.

This book provides simple methods to prevent and treat pressure ulcers. The reader will have a toolbox to use to truly understand pressure ulcers. Evidence-based strategies will be noted as well as practical measures, not simply textbook findings. These measures will include important prevention mechanisms; how to identify, detect, and assess pressure ulcers; and basic treatment modalities that can be used in any setting.

Mary Ellen Dziedzic

The Basics of Pressure Ulcers

The Problem of
Pressure Ulcer Occurrence

Pressure ulcers can cause patients serious harm and can affect their ability to function. Caused by pressure most often over a bony prominence, these ulcers can cause serious infection and require plastic surgery as well as long-term intervention. Chronic ulcers can take months to years to heal and may require long-term nursing care. It is therefore important for the nurse to understand how pressure ulcers occur, to have a clear means of identification, and to understand why prevention is necessary.

Upon completion of this chapter, the reader will be able to:

1. Define and properly describe pressure ulcers
2. Discuss current staging and identification guidelines
3. Identify the importance of prevention as it is related to the cost of pressure ulcer care

WHAT IS A PRESSURE ULCER?

Before pressure ulcers can be cared for or prevented, it is first necessary to understand what they are. Pressure ulcers, also called decubitus ulcers or bed sores, are essentially that—*pressure* ulcers. Once this fact is understood, everything else required for assessment and treatment will fall into place. According to the International National Pressure Ulcer Advisory Panel (NPUAP)–European Pressure Ulcer Advisory Panel (EPUAP) Pressure Ulcer Classification System (2009): "A pressure ulcer is a localized injury to the skin and/or underlying tissue usually over a bony prominence, as a result of pressure or pressure in combination with shear. A number of contributing or confounding factors are associated with pressure ulcers; the significance of these factors is yet to be elucidated." When analyzed this makes sense: Bones protruding at these sites cause pressure to the skin and tissue; when a person is positioned on these areas for a period of time (often 2 hours or less; EPUAP and NPUAP, 2009), damage to tissue above the bone can occur simply because of the person's body weight. This is truly *pressure* and is how a pressure ulcer can begin.

═══════════════════*FAST FACTS in a NUTSHELL*

Injury to the skin and underlying tissue most commonly occurs at the sacrum, ischium, heel, or trochanter (Wound Ostomy and Continence Nurses Society, 2006–2011). Positioning patients so that pressure is off these sites is important to prevention.

Essentially all pressure ulcers are caused by pressure of some sort, whether internal, external, or from a medical or personal device. Shear, friction, and moisture do play a part in the development of pressure ulcers. These forces alone or in combination can cause tissue damage.

Friction

Friction occurs when two forces rub together (Sibbald, 2011); for example, when a patient with heavy thighs increases the amount of walking or running on a hot day. Think about the rubbing and the red raw appearance of the skin on the inner thighs; that is from friction. Friction causes skin damage and usually alone does not cause pressure ulcers but can in combination with other forces.

Shear

Shear is defined as the applied force that can cause an opposite, parallel sliding motion in the planes of an object. Shear is affected by the amount of pressure that is exerted on the underlying tissue (Wound Ostomy and Continence Nurses Society, 2006–2011). An example is a patient in a wheelchair who slips out of the chair. Damage to the skin often occurs to the posterior thighs: Skin is soft, the chair is not, and bone is not. Such forces can cause damage, especially over time. This type of damage is often evident from thigh to knee where the skin can actually become sheared. Another common area where shear can occur is when a patient is sitting in bed with the head elevated to the highest level. The body often slips down. Here damage often occurs to the sacrum or heel of the foot.

═══════════════════════════════ *FAST FACTS in a NUTSHELL*

When a patient sits in bed with the head above a 30-degree angle, serious skin injury can occur to the sacrum and heels. This position should be reserved for meals and the patient lowered as soon as possible. If the patient's head must remain above 30 degrees for medical reasons, it is important to reposition the patient frequently to decrease the pressure on soft tissue.

Moisture

Moisture itself causes tissue damage and can lead to pressure ulcers in combination with the other forces of shear and friction. A patient's skin can be moist from perspiration, incontinence of bowel and bladder, and external moisture such as from leaking intravenous fluids, drainage from wounds, and leaking tubes. Moisture changes the balance of the skin, removing protective oils. If the moisture is acidic—such as from incontinence or other body fluid—damage can occur even in a brief amount of time. Bowel incontinence is one of the highest predictors in patients for developing pressure ulcers in the home (Bergquist-Beringer, 2011). Again moisture alone does not cause a pressure ulcer; moisture in combination with the above forces can cause a pressure ulcer.

This may seem confusing. Simple incontinence causing dermatitis can be improved by adding a toileting regimen or a consistent use of a barrier cream. When there is pressure and moisture, serious damage to the skin and underlying structures can occur. Moisture is an important concept in preventing pressure ulcers and skin damage and will be discussed in more detail in upcoming chapters.

CURRENT STAGING GUIDELINES: NPUAP-EPUAP

The first step in understanding pressure ulcers is to identify them. Pressure ulcers are most often graded or staged based on severity. The term "staging" might commonly mean that something must go through stages—as a caterpillar to a butterfly. Not true with pressure ulcers. An ulcer is staged on specific characteristics of the ulcer. Ulcers, like the human body, do not follow a specific pattern or gradient (Sibbald, 2011). Just as human beings are different, pressure ulcers are different.

The International NPUAP-EPUAP Pressure Ulcer Classification System (2009) is the most widely accepted classification system for identifying pressure ulcers and provides a simple means of identifying the severity of pressure ulcers. The key to identification of an ulcer's severity is to clearly match the characteristics to those of the classification system. Classifying ulcers is not black and white and nurses often differ on how an ulcer is staged; it is therefore important to focus on current evidence.

Following is the International NPUAP-EPUAP Pressure Ulcer Classification System. (Used with permission, photos courtesy of Convatec.)

Category/Stage I: Nonblanchable Erythema

Category/Stage I involves intact skin with nonblanchable redness of a localized area usually over a bony prominence (Figure 1.1). Darkly pigmented skin may not have visible blanching; its color may differ from the surrounding area.

The area may be painful, firm soft, warmer or cooler as compared to adjacent tissue. Category/Stage I may be difficult to detect in individuals with dark skin tones. May indicate "at risk" persons (a heralding sign of risk).

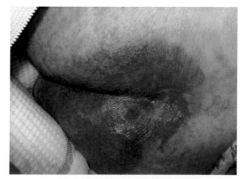

FIGURE 1.1
Category/Stage I ulcer.
Source: National
Pressure Ulcer Advisory
Panel Resources.

Category/Stage II: Partial Thickness Skin Loss

Partial thickness loss of dermis presenting as a shallow open ulcer with a red-pink wound bed, without slough. May also present as an intact or open/ruptured serum-filled blister.

Presents as a shiny or dry shallow ulcer without slough or bruising (Figure 1.2). This category/stage should not be used to describe skin tears, tape burns, perineal dermatitis, maceration, or excoriation. Bruising indicates suspected deep tissue injury.

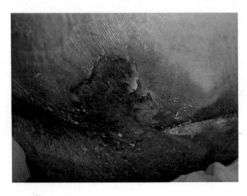

FIGURE 1.2
Category/Stage II ulcer.
Source: National Pressure Ulcer Advisory Panel Resources.

Category/Stage III: Full Thickness Skin Loss

In full thickness tissue loss, subcutaneous fat may be visible but bone, tendon, or muscle is not exposed. Slough may be present but does not obscure the depth of tissue loss. It may include undermining or tunneling.

The depth of a Category/Stage III pressure ulcer varies by anatomical location (Figure 1.3). The bridge of the nose, ear, occiput, and malleolus do not have subcutaneous issue and Category/Stage III ulcers can be shallow. In contrast, areas of significant adiposity can develop extremely deep Category/Stage III pressure ulcers. Bone/tendon is not visible or directly palpable.

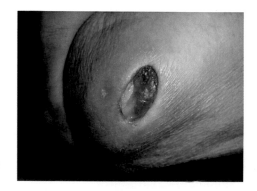

FIGURE 1.3
Category/Stage III
ulcer.
Source: National
Pressure Ulcer Advisory
Panel Resources.

Category/Stage IV: Full Thickness Tissue Loss

Category IV is full thickness tissue loss with exposed bone, tendon, or muscle. Slough or eschar may be present on some parts of the wound bed. It often includes undermining or tunneling.

The depth of a Category/Stage IV pressure ulcer varies by anatomical location (Figure 1.4). The bridge of the nose, ear, occiput, and malleolus do not have subcutaneous tissue and these ulcers can be shallow. Category/Stage IV ulcers can extend to muscle and/or supporting structures (e.g., fascia, tendon, or joint capsule) making osteomyelitis possible. Exposed bone/tendon is visible or directly palpable.

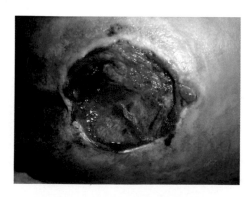

FIGURE 1.4
Category/Stage IV
ulcer.
Source: National
Pressure Ulcer Advisory
Panel Resources.

Unstageable: Depth Unknown

This is full thickness tissue loss in which the base of the ulcer is covered by slough (yellow, tan, gray, green, or brown) and/or eschar (tan, brown, or black) in the wound bed.

Until enough slough and/or eschar is removed or exposed, the base of the wound, the true depth, and, therefore, the category/stage cannot be determined (Figure 1.5). Stable (dry, adherent, intact without erythema or fluctuance) eschar on the heels serves as "the body's natural (biological) cover" and should not be removed.

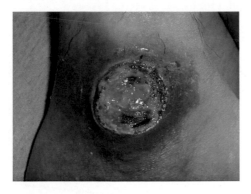

FIGURE 1.5
Unstageable ulcer.
Source: National Pressure Ulcer Advisory Panel Resources.

Suspected Deep Tissue Injury: Depth Unknown

This is a purple- or maroon-colored localized area of discolored, intact skin or blood-filled blister due to damage of underlying soft tissue from pressure and/or shear (Figure 1.6). The area may be preceded by tissue that is painful, firm, mushy, boggy, and warmer or cooler as compared to adjacent tissue.

Deep tissue injury may be difficult to detect in individuals with dark skin tones. Evolution may include a thin blister over a dark wound bed. The wound may further evolve and become covered by thin eschar. Evolution may be rapid, exposing additional layers of tissue even with optimal treatment.

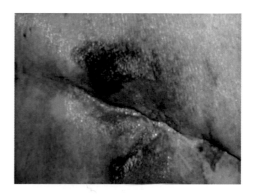

FIGURE 1.6
Suspected deep tissue
injury.
Source: National
Pressure Ulcer Advisory
Panel Resources.

Pressure ulcers are not back staged; that is, as they heal they do not become a Stage II from a Stage III. The ulcer is then always a Stage III; a healing Stage III will fill in with granulation tissue but not muscle. When the patient has a suspected deep tissue injury, the results may be devastating. The damage can be bone deep even though it may appear as ecchymotic to the untrained eye. That is why it is important to clearly identify and quickly act to prevent further damage and to treat what is already there (Sibbald, 2011). The rest of this book focuses on additional tools for assessing risk for pressure ulcer development, tips for prevention and care, treatment, and finally the development of a pressure ulcer prevention program.

TIPS FOR IDENTIFICATION OF PRESSURE ULCERS

The skin is the largest organ of the body and organs can fail. It is therefore important to conduct a thorough skin survey not only on admission, but also with every patient contact. Every time you assist a patient with basic care, inspect the skin for changes. When you help a patient to the toilet, dress, bathe, transfer, and/or position the patient, take the opportunity to check and provide skin care. Skin assessment will be discussed in more detail later in this book but skin inspection should be conducted routinely and in a specific time frame—for example, every 8 hours.

An important aspect in identifying skin issues is to become attuned to changes. A pressure area is obviously different from surrounding skin. Skin may be red because of irritation or moisture but if the area does not fade when touched and then released (blanching), this may be an indication of a Stage I pressure ulcer.

For people with darker skin, the skin may look darker or lighter than the surrounding skin. Skin may look red, purple, or blue in color. Become accustomed to feeling a patient's skin especially if a change is noted. Feel the temperature of the skin; just as with the appearance, the temperature may be different in the problem area. It may be cooler or warmer. In addition to temperature, a pressure ulcer may feel firmer, raised, or boggy (spongy). When an area of pressure is noted, feel for changes (University of Texas School of Nursing, n.d.).

Skin inspection is done from head to toe. Step by step, carefully look at all parts of the patient:

- Check the head for pressure areas from lying in one position.
- Assess ears, nose, cheeks, and chin especially if the person tends to favor one side when in bed.
- Check the shoulders, scapula, and elbows.
- Look at the fingers and hands if the patient clenches the fingers.
- Look at the hips, buttocks, sacrum, and abdomen.
- Check under folds, and look in the gluteal cleft as ulcers often occur at the coccyx or a split may occur due to moisture and incorrect movement.
- Carefully look at the thighs, groin, perianal area, and behind and between the knees.

- Look at the heels by actually lifting the leg to visualize or use a mirror. Touch can be important for heels as the heel may feel soft, boggy, or blistered.
- Finally check the bottoms and tops of the feet, toes, and between the toes if they rub together.

═══════════════════════════════════*FAST FACTS in a NUTSHELL*

When checking a patient's skin for pressure ulcers or other problems, it is important to be thorough and consistent. This is an area where continuity of nursing care plays an important role. Subtle changes can then readily be detected.

When doing a careful skin inspection, remember to look at areas that are under clothing or equipment. Clothing can be constricting and the patient may not even be aware. This can occur often in the groin, feet, or at the waist. In addition, if a tube is allowed to lie between skin folds or on the skin for prolonged periods, pressure ulcers can occur. For example, a urinary catheter can cause an ulcer in the labia.

THE COST OF PRESSURE ULCER CARE

It is clear that skin care is an important part of a patient's care. Pressure ulcers can be devastating to patients and families. If the pressure ulcer is significant it can cause infection, often to the bone (osteomyelitis). This type of infection can require expensive treatment, surgery, long-term hospitalization, prolonged rehabilitation, and sometimes amputation of the affected part or death. Every part of a patient's life can be affected.

Pressure ulcer care is expensive. In the United States, these ulcers cost over $1 billion annually and add an additional $2.2 million Medicare hospital days to the United States health care system. The cost of treatment can be anywhere from $6,000 to $60,000 depending on the stage. Some sources indicate that the cost of care per ulcer can be up to $90,000. Plastic and reconstructive surgery for pressure ulcers can cost $25,000 or more per patient (Wake, 2010). These costs alone indicate the importance of pressure ulcer prevention and care. Add the human suffering factor and the importance of prevention becomes even more significant.

This book focuses on pressure ulcer identification, care, and prevention. The next section reviews the anatomy, physiology, and pathophysiology of the skin to assist in further understanding pressure ulcer development.

2

Anatomy, Physiology, and Pathophysiology of the Skin

Skin is the largest organ of the body, providing the body with protection, immunity, thermoregulation, sensation, metabolism, and communication. Weighing at least 6 pounds or 15% of the total body weight, skin essentially provides a protective barrier from the external environment and maintains homeostasis in the internal environment. Unlike other organs, the skin can regenerate and can withstand limited chemical and physical assaults. The appearance of a person's skin is a key indicator of the person's health status (Goodwin, 2011). With these facts in hand, understanding why pressure ulcers occur is to understand the skin itself.

Upon completion of this chapter, the reader will be able to:

1. Identify the key functions of the skin
2. Discuss the anatomy and physiology of the skin
3. Understand how pressure affects skin, causing a pressure ulcer

FUNCTION OF THE SKIN

It was already noted that the skin is the largest organ of the body. The average adult has over 20 square feet of skin, thickest at the souls of the feet and thinnest at the eyelids and tips of the ears. Changes in the skin often indicate illness or other issues within the body.

There are three layers of the skin that will be discussed: the dermis, epidermis, and subcutaneous tissues. These layers are responsible for seven major functions:

1. Prevention of the loss of fluid and electrolytes to maintain the internal environment
2. Protection of the skin from external agents
3. Regulation of body temperature
4. Self-maintenance and wound repair
5. Vitamin D production
6. Provision of the sensations of touch, temperature, and pain
7. Delayed reaction to foreign substances

The skin provides essential protection from the external environment. It is a barrier to chemical, physical, and biological assaults. The skin is continuous with the mucous membrane lining the skin throughout. If there is an assault to the integrity of the skin, the protection provided is compromised (Goodwin, 2011).

FAST FACTS in a NUTSHELL

Because the skin provides such key functions to the body, protection of the skin is important. Moisturizing and barrier creams are important tools in protecting the balance of the skin.

ANATOMY AND PHYSIOLOGY OF THE SKIN

The skin is composed of three layers: the dermis, epidermis, and subcutaneous tissue (or hypodermis), each having specific functions (Figure 2.1).

Epidermis

The outermost layer, the epidermis is an epithelium layer composed of two major cell types: keratinocytes and dendritic cells. The majority of cells are keratinocytes. These cells form a barrier against environmental assault of pathogens, heat, UV radiation, and water loss. The dendritic cells are essentially the messengers between the innate and adaptive immunity.

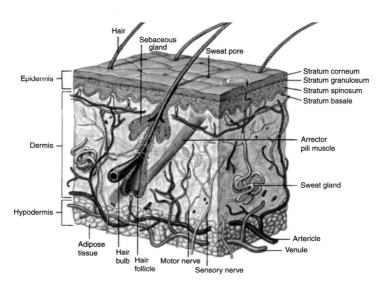

FIGURE 2.1 Physiology of the skin.
Source: www.convatec.com. ConvatecUSA. Skin and Skin Care.

The epidermis is then broken down into four layers. The basal cell layer (stratum germinativum), the squamous cell layer (stratum spinosum), the granular layer (stratum granulosum), and the cornified or horny cell layer (stratum corneum). This layer is constantly renewing, with the basal cells undergoing proliferation to renew the outermost epidermis. The epidermis is a dynamic tissue; it is in constant motion and maintains a constant number of cells. Epidermal cells morph and differentiate, which is somewhat regulated by the dermis but mostly by the cells themselves. The dermal–epidermal junction is an interface between the epidermis and dermis. It is formed by the basement membrane, which is porous. It is here that there is an exchange of fluids and cells (Goodwin, 2011).

═══════════════════════════════════*FAST FACTS in a NUTSHELL*

If the balance of the epidermis is disrupted and there is a constant thickening of the epidermis, conditions such as psoriasis can erupt. If cell death (apoptosis = programmed cell death) is not regulated, tumors of the skin can occur.

Dermis

The dermis makes up most of the skin providing elasticity, pliability, and tensile strength. Because of this strength, it protects the body from mechanical injury, and assists in binding water and in thermoregulation. It is here that there is a matrix of components, primarily elastin and collagen. The dermis and epidermis interact while maintaining the integrity of both tissues. This interaction is important in wound healing (Goodwin, 2011). The structures found in the dermis are the nerve and sensory fibers, hair follicles, sebaceous glands, and sweat glands. The atypical layers of the dermis are folded to form dermal papillae that are prominent in thick skin.

The blood supply of the dermis occurs in the junctions within the dermis and the lower portion of the dermal–subcutaneous interface. The dermal papillae are supplied by capillaries and arterioles in the superficial plexus. The larger blood vessels supply the deeper plexus. A large number of nerve bundles along with the smaller blood vessels are found in the dermis. This blood supply is also important to wound healing and in pressure ulcer prevention. If the blood supply is diminished as in any body part, that part can become damaged or die.

Hypodermis

Subcutaneous fat or hypodermis is the storehouse of energy. It is considered an endocrine organ. It provides protection to the body and maintains its homeostasis along with the other layers. It slows heat loss by providing a layer of insulation between the inner and external environment.

Maintaining skin integrity is important to health. Normally skin is elastic and lubricated and slightly acidic. This protective mantle protects the skin from the growth of pathogens. In addition, Langerhans cells, which are part of the cell network, also prevent infections. All of these functions are important to wound healing.

THE BASICS OF WOUND HEALING

Nonhealing or chronic wounds are wounds that do not progress through the normal phases of healing. The wound is essentially stalled, which can be caused by internal or external factors. Wound healing is complex and requires restoration of the tissue layers and cellular structures. There are two types of wounds:

- *Acute wounds*: Caused by surgical intervention or trauma. They follow the normal healing process.
- *Chronic wounds*: Healing takes longer and wounds do not progress through the predicable stages of healing. These are wounds that are essentially not resolved.

Wounds heal in three ways:

- *Primary intention:* The wound edges are approximated and are held together by surgical methods such as staples or sutures. Healing occurs by epithelialization and connective tissue attachments. The cells migrate and heal the wound.
- *Secondary intention:* Used most often in infected surgical wounds, trauma, or wounds caused by chronic injury or diseases. The wound edges are not approximated and healing occurs through the development of granulation tissue, contraction of wound edges, and then epithelialization. This tissue is the only regeneration that occurs, as muscle and other structures do not regenerate. Wounds like this are said to heal from the bottom up.
- *Tertiary intention:* Wounds are left open usually to restart granulation and provide treatment and then closed in a surgical method.

Wounds go through a series of phases from initial injury to final closure. The three phases of wound healing are:

Inflammatory phase: This phase begins with the initial injury and ends with clot formation. Cells migrate to the wound, forming clots. Cytokines and platelet-derived growth factors are brought to the injury. Here cellular growth and formation are influenced. The inflammatory phase progresses through hemostasis and inflammation.

- *Hemostasis:* In hemostasis the vasculature response is to control bleeding; this phase lasts only a few hours. Platelets aggregate, initiating a temporary barrier to infection. In this phase vasoconstriction occurs along with thromboplastic production.
- *Inflammation:* In this stage the body attempts to clean the wound of debris. Vasodilation occurs, resulting in leakage of plasma, neutrophils, and cytokines into surrounding tissue. This is noted as edema and heat around the wound.

Proliferative phase: This phase is longer lasting, usually 2 days to up to 3 weeks. It begins by the filling in of the wound with granulation tissue. Here connective tissue is stimulated. After the wound is filled with granulation tissue, the wound edges begin epithelialization. This starts from the outside edges and progresses toward the center of the wound.

Remodeling phase: The body continues to heal after a wound is closed. This phase can take up to 3 years if the patient has comorbidities such as diabetes. The wound matrix is changed and the collagen increases the strength of the tissues (Broderick, 2009).

════════════════════════════*FAST FACTS in a NUTSHELL*

After scar formation and remodeling, the area is prone to re-injury or breakdown as this skin is not as strong as uncompromised skin. If a patient had a significant pressure ulcer, that area can be easily harmed. Protection is therefore always important.

PATHOPHYSIOLOGY OF PRESSURE ULCERS

The factors causing pressure ulcers are separated into two major groups:

- *Intrinsic:* Factors from within the body such as disease/comorbidities, medications, poor nutrition, age, dehydration/fluid status, poor mobility, incontinence, suppleness, and weight.
- *Extrinsic:* The external influences that cause skin damage or changes such as pressure, shear, friction, or moisture.

These factors put stress on the skin, causing it to fail. Capillaries and arterioles within the skin are important to provide the skin with viability and oxygenation. The average mean capillary pressure equals about 17 mmHg and any external pressures exceeding this will cause capillary obstruction. Tissues that are dependent on these capillaries are deprived of their blood supply. Eventually the tissue will become ischemic and die (Waterlow, 2009). This is what happens when there is pressure on a bony prominence for prolonged periods. The blood supply is diminished and the area above the pressure does not get sufficient oxygen and dies.

Shearing forces will only exist if pressure, usually caused by the person's own body weight, is also present. Shearing forces occur when a part of the body tries to move but the surface of the skin remains fixed. Shear alone does not cause a pressure ulcer but may cause the epidermis or dermis to slough as in a skin tear. Shear in combination with friction, pressure, or moisture causes a pressure ulcer. Friction is actually caused by the body's resistance to movement and causes increased pressure in combination with shear.

Moist skin from perspiration and incontinence in combination with the other forces can cause a pressure ulcer. Moisture also can cause the skin to become macerated. This type of skin appears moist, often white and frail. Macerated skin also is more susceptible to friction and shear. Moist skin is different than incontinent-associated skin damage. Such damage occurs because of the high caustic nature of urine and feces. The damage can be devastating but is not the same as a pressure ulcer and will be discussed in more detail in later chapters.

It is evident that pressure ulcers are caused by multiple factors. The damage caused to skin and delicate tissues can be devastating. It is much less expensive to prevent the damage than to treat it. The rest of this book will focus on assessment, prevention, and treatment.

3

Risk Assessment

Pressure ulcers present a health risk to all types of patients. Patients who are debilitated because of hospital admission, chronic disease, or age are at particular risk for pressure ulcer development simply because of their health status. While it may be assumed that highly skilled clinical nurses would be adept at assessing a patient's risk for developing pressure ulcers, several studies indicate that use of a valid instrument is much better at predicting risk (Pajula & Osborn, 2008). Use of these tools can provide the evidence and validation needed for outside agencies including the Centers for Medicare and Medicaid Services (CMS) to appropriately reimburse for the care of pressure ulcers, as the cost can be very high.

Upon completion of this chapter, the reader will be able to:

1. Define what is meant by assessing a patient's risk for pressure ulcer development
2. Discuss the importance of risk assessment to pressure ulcer prevention and successfully utilize a risk assessment tool to identify patients that may develop pressure ulcers
3. Identify the importance of careful initial assessment and identification of ulcers that are present on admission

ASSESSING A PATIENT'S RISK FOR PRESSURE ULCER DEVELOPMENT

What Is Risk Assessment?

Assessing risk for pressure ulcer development is an important tool in pressure ulcer prevention. Even ambulatory patients may be at high risk for pressure ulcer development. Some risk factors include age, altered sensory perception, altered mental status, impaired circulation, comorbid conditions such as diabetes, long length of stay at an acute- or long-term care facility, or complicated surgical procedures (Kottner & Dassen, 2010).

Risk identification is multifaceted and can be made simple by using one of the tools discussed in this section. Identifying patients at risk is an important first step toward planning the intensity of and the implementation of appropriate prevention interventions.

Why Is It Important to Assess a Patient's Risk?

Assessing a patient's pressure ulcer risk helps guide implementation of appropriate nursing care designed to halt pressure ulcers from developing. When used correctly, the information obtained provides a picture of the patient's overall health status and the strategies that need to be implemented to prevent skin breakdown. Some key identifiers include:

- What is the patient's general health appearance?
- How mobile is the person? Is movement easy or difficult?
- Is the patient incontinent?
- Are there other issues with moisture?
- Is friction or shear a problem for the patient?

All these factors are important not only to preventing skin breakdown but in the total care of the patient.

===============================*FAST FACTS in a NUTSHELL*

Risk assessment tools are used on a regular basis. They are most effective when used consistently and often (every shift in acute care, every day or two times weekly in a longer-care facility, and every visit in home care). The use of the tool really does paint a picture of the patient's well-being in terms that everyone can understand.

Risk Assessment Scales

Several scales are commonly used in health care settings. The three more commonly used and more familiar scales are the Norton Scale, the Waterlow Scale, and the Braden Scale (Wake, 2010). Each uses subscales to determine an individual risk score. Though the scales do not overlap, many of the assessment categories used in the scales are similar.

The Norton Scale

The Norton Scale was created in England in 1962 and was the first pressure ulcer risk evaluation tool. The scale focuses on physical condition, mental condition, activity, mobility, and incontinence. The tool is used widely especially in long-term care ("Norton Pressure Score," 1962). The tool is somewhat subjective in that it requires the user to make judgments to determine good, fair, poor, and very bad. There is no accounting for nutrition.

The Waterlow Scale

The Waterlow Scale was designed in 1985 by Judy Waterlow while working as a clinical nurse teacher. The tool was originally designed for use by students. The subscales of this work include body build and weight, skin type, sex and age, malnutrition screening continence, and mobility. In addition there are special considerations that include tissue malnutrition, neurological deficit, and major surgery or trauma (Waterlow, 1985, revised 2005).

The Braden Scale

The Braden Scale for Predicting Pressure Sore Risk is an evidence-based tool for predicting pressure ulcer risk. It was developed in 1998 by Barbara Braden and Nancy Bergstrom and is based on their extensive research in patient care. This tool is the one most commonly used and has been scientifically validated. The Braden Scale shows optimal validation and the best sensitivity/specificity balance (57.1%/67.5%, respectively); its score is a good pressure ulcer risk predictor (odds ratio = 4.08, 95% confidence interval [CI] = 2.56–6.48) (Pajula & Osborn, 2008).

The scale is a simple tool and can be used in all settings (Table 3.1). It is a rating scale made up of six subscales scored from 1 to 4, for total scores that range from 6 to 23. The lower score indicates a lower level of function and patient status and as a result a higher level of risk for pressure ulcer development. A score of 19 or higher would indicate that the patient is at low risk, with little need for intervention at this time (Braden, 1998). This score is usually done on admission to a facility or agency. It is also done periodically in acute care, usually every shift or every 24 hours and adjusted based on changes in patient condition. It is used in other areas on a regular and consistent basis.

TABLE 3.1 Braden Pressure Ulcer Risk Assessment

Patient's Name _____ **Evaluator's Name** _____ **Date of Assessment** _____

Sensory Perception Ability to respond meaningfully to pressure-related discomfort	**1. Completely Limited** Unresponsive (does not moan, flinch, or gasp) to painful stimuli, due to diminished level of consciousness or sedation OR limited ability to feel pain over most of body surface.	**2. Very Limited** Responds only to painful stimuli. Cannot communicate discomfort except by moaning or restlessness OR has a sensory impairment which limits the ability to feel pain or discomfort over 1/2 of body.	**3. Slightly Limited** Responds to verbal commands, but cannot always communicate discomfort or need to be turned OR has some sensory impairment which limits ability to feel pain or discomfort in one or two extremities.	**4. No Impairment** Responds to verbal commands, has no sensory deficit which would limit ability to feel or voice pain or discomfort.
Moisture Degree to which skin is exposed to moisture	**1. Constantly Moist** Skin is kept moist almost constantly by perspiration, urine, etc. Dampness is detected every time patient is moved or turned.	**2. Very Moist** Skin is often, but not always, moist. Linen must be changed at least once a shift.	**3. Occasionally Moist** Skin is occasionally moist, requiring an extra linen change approximately once a day.	**4. Rarely Moist** Skin is usually dry, linen only requires changing at routine intervals.
Activity Degree of physical activity	**1. Bedfast** Confined to bed.	**2. Chairfast** Ability to walk severely limited or nonexistent. Cannot bear weight and/or must be assisted into chair or wheelchair.	**3. Walks Occasionally** Walks occasionally during day, but for very short distances, with or without assistance. Spends majority of each shift in bed or chair.	**4. Walks Frequently** Walks outside the room at least twice a day and inside room at least once every 2 hours during waking hours.
Mobility Ability to change and control body position	**1. Completely Immobile** Does not make even slight changes in body or extremity position without assistance.	**2. Very Limited** Makes occasional slight changes in body or extremity position but unable to make frequent or significant changes independently.	**3. Slightly Limited** Makes frequent though slight changes in body or extremity position independently.	**4. No Limitations** Makes major and frequent changes in position without assistance.

(continued)

29

TABLE 3.1 Braden Pressure Ulcer Risk Assessment (continued)

Patient's Name _____ Evaluator's Name _____ Date of Assessment _____

	1. Very Poor	2. Probably Inadequate	3. Adequate	4. Excellent
Nutrition Usual food intake pattern	Never eats a complete meal. Rarely eats more than 1/3 of any food offered. Eats 2 servings or less of protein (meat or dairy products) per day. Takes fluids poorly. Does not take a liquid dietary supplement OR is NPO and/or maintained on clear liquids or IVs for more than 5 days.	Rarely eats a complete meal and generally eats only about 1/2 of any food offered. Protein intake includes only 3 servings of meat or dairy products per day. Occasionally will take a dietary supplement OR receives less than optimum amount of liquid diet or tube feeding.	Eats over half of most meals. Eats a total of 4 servings of protein (meat, dairy products) each day. Occasionally will refuse a meal, but will usually take a supplement if offered OR is on a tube feeding or TPN regimen which probably meets most of nutritional needs.	Eats most of every meal. Never refuses a meal. Usually eats a total of 4 or more servings of meat and dairy products. Occasionally eats between meals. Does not require supplementation.
	1. Problem	2. Potential Problem	3. No Apparent Problem	
Friction and Shear	Requires moderate to maximum assistance in moving. Complete lifting without sliding against sheets is impossible. Frequently slides down in bed or chair, requiring frequent repositioning with maximum assistance. Spasticity, contractures, or agitation leads to almost constant friction.	Moves feebly or requires minimum assistance. During a move, skin probably slides to some extent against sheets, chair, restraints, or other devices. Maintains relatively good position in chair or bed most of the time but occasionally slides down.	Moves in bed and in chair independently and has sufficient muscle strength to lift up completely during move. Maintains good position in bed or chair at all times.	

The use of a scale such as the Braden Scale for Predicting Pressure Sore Risk is part of a prevention program and is most successful when all nurses within the facility are trained in its use and utilize it on a regular basis. The CMS requires that a valid tool for pressure ulcer prevention be utilized on admission and repeated on a consistent and regular basis. This benefits the patient as it facilitates optimal care, the facility receives appropriate reimbursement for the care provided, and nursing staff are relieved of the intensive treatment required to care for late-stage pressure ulcers (CMS, 2012).

It must be noted that a patient may have additional risk factors not indicated by a pressure ulcer risk scale. Patients who are having surgery, for example, have additional needs, as they are subject to immobility, may be dehydrated, or have poor nutrition due to nothing-by-mouth status. Postoperative patients may appear well and able to change position easily but may not do so due to postoperative pain. Pain then becomes the risk and effective pain management the intervention. Young and essentially healthy people do develop pressure ulcers when their bodies are under stress. It is important to be aware of these factors and use prevention tools for these patients as well (He, Liu, & Chen, 2012).

THE IMPORTANCE OF IDENTIFYING PRESSURE ULCERS PRESENT ON ADMISSION

The CMS is most often the primary payer for health care facilities. Health care agencies rely heavily on this reimbursement. Facilities that do not cultivate other payer sources can quickly have financial difficulties. In terms of pressure ulcer reporting, the CMS has made it clear that reimbursement is affected if serious ulcers (Stage III or IV) occur in a health care facility. According to CMS guidelines, as of October 1, 2008, hospitals will not receive reimbursement for specific patient safety issues, such as pressure ulcers, that occurred in that hospital. The case would be paid as if the secondary diagnosis were not present. If a patient had a stroke, barring complications the hospital would receive approximately $6,000 for the patient's care and $8,000 if there were a Stage III ulcer identified as present on admission. If the ulcer was not identified as present on admission, then that money is subtracted (Healthcare Cost and Utilization Project [HCUP], 2011).

Reimbursement for hospitals and now other facilities can be seriously affected if pressure ulcers—Stage III or Stage IV—are not identified as present on admission. It is, therefore, important that findings on the initial patient assessment are clearly documented. In general, a patient admission assessment is done within the first 8 hours of care but not beyond 24 hours. Pressure ulcers can occur quickly; CMS guidelines indicate that if it is past 24 hours, the ulcer occurred in the current facility. The lack of documentation can seriously affect the amount of reimbursement received.

ENSURING REIMBURSEMENT FOR ULCER CARE

General Reporting Requirements

A present on admission or POA indicator is required for all claims involving Medicare inpatient admissions to acute care hospitals. POA is defined as "present at the time the order for inpatient admission occurs—conditions that develop during an outpatient encounter, including emergency department, observation, or outpatient surgery, are considered POA" (CMS, 2012). The POA indicator involves secondary and primary diagnoses.

Inconsistent, missing, conflicting, or unclear documentation must be resolved by the provider before a claim will be paid.

Based on the above findings, the importance of consistent, complete documentation in the medical record is necessary when caring for a patient with pressure ulcers that are present on admission. The CMS indicates that medical record documentation from any provider that participates in the care of the patient may be used to support the determination of whether a condition was present on admission. In the context of the official coding guidelines, the term "provider" means a physician or any qualified health care practitioner who is legally accountable for establishing the patient's diagnosis (CMS, 2012).

FAST FACTS in a NUTSHELL

Everyone caring for a patient with pressure ulcers needs to be on the same page. Nursing and physician documentation should mirror each other. It is clear that education and communication are needed at all levels to ensure present on admission is documented.

In acute care there are very ill patients, especially those in critical care. This is where clear documentation of the patient's condition is very important, not only in the care of the patient but for appropriate payment. Often patients in intensive care can develop serious ulcers. Based on their condition, medications, treatment, and prognosis, often these ulcers can be identified as unavoidable. According to the Wound Ostomy and Continence Nurses Society, the burden of illness is so overwhelming that even with the best prevention methods pressure ulcers can still occur. The skin is the largest organ of the body and organs can fail (Wound Ostomy and Continence Nurses Society, 2009).

Patients themselves can be their own worst enemies. Patients often refuse care even with appropriate education concerning the need for prevention interventions. It is up to the caregiver to make every effort to encourage the patient to participate in prevention methods. However, some patients will continue to refuse. Documentation with these patients is of the utmost importance. Clearly document the education, the intervention attempts, and every time the patient refuses care. Including family members in the education may also be necessary. Sometimes patients may not be fully able to make those decisions on their own, so others may need to be involved.

Activities aimed at pressure ulcer prevention are often necessary for most patients. Patients who appear well may actually need intervention to move or reposition. If pain is an issue for a patient, pain will have to be controlled as much as possible in order for the patient to move comfortably. Patients who are critically ill still need preventions such as repositioning (even slight shifts in position can produce sufficient off-loading for tissues). The following chapters will focus on further patient assessment as it relates to pressure ulcers.

4

Back to Basics in Skin Care and Assessment

Nursing, according to Florence Nightingale, reflects "the activities that promote health which occur in any caregiving situation." The goal of nursing is to have the patient achieve the best possible condition for nature to act. Altering the individual's environment can promote health. This is nursing care at its simplest and it is very pertinent to the discussion of skin care. Without basic skin care, health cannot be established and the skin can fail (Skretkowicz, 2010).

Upon completion of this chapter, the reader will be able to:

1. Discuss Florence Nightingale's concepts as they relate to the care of patients' skin
2. Identify evidence-based methods to conduct a thorough skin assessment
3. Apply basic concepts of pressure ulcer prevention when caring for patients

APPLYING NIGHTINGALE'S PHILOSOPHY OF HEALTH

The major concepts about health articulated by Nightingale that were related to the environment included *ventilation and warming, light and noise, cleanliness, health in houses and bed and bedding, personal cleanliness, variety, offering hope and advice, food, and observation* (Skretkowicz, 2010). Each of these concepts affects the patient's environment and the environment of the patient's skin. Most skin care recommendations are a result of expert opinion and consensus. It is clear that if a patient is left dirty, with poor ventilation, and without proper nutrition, the patient becomes unhealthy and develops skin issues and disease as a result (Lyder, 2008). Using Nightingale's concepts can help put skin care in perspective.

INTERVENTIONS TO MAINTAIN HEALTH

Humidifying the Environment

Artificial air from heating units and air conditioning may contribute to dry skin, which is especially detrimental to the elderly patient. Providing moist and humidified air is important to help prevent skin from cracking and peeling, especially during winter months. Skin does change with age; it thins and flattens due to a decrease in fatty tissue and a decrease in tissue moisture. Dry skin, therefore, is common in more than 70% of nursing home patients. Elderly people experience dry flaky skin on their extremities, heels, and elbows (Hess, 2008). When moisture is lost, skin can become irritated and inflamed, which can lead to further skin damage. Scaling and dryness are directly related to pressure ulcer development ("Pressure Ulcer," *The New York Times Health Guide,* 2013). Intact, moisturized skin decreases the chance of pressure ulcer development. To increase the humidity, it may be necessary to use a room humidifier especially for people in the home environment with very dry or cracking skin.

Light

Light is another concept noted by Nightingale that impacts health and, consequently, the health of the skin. Ultraviolet (UV) light in small amounts is beneficial and necessary for the production of vitamin D and the absorption of calcium (World Health Organization [WHO], 2013). Vitamin D increases calcium and phosphorus absorption from food and plays an important role in skeletal development, immune functions, and blood cell formation. Also, UV radiation under medical supervision is used to treat several diseases such as rickets, psoriasis, eczema, and jaundice. At the same time, it is important to note that the sun does cause degenerative changes in the skin, blood vessels, and connective tissue, and prolonged exposure has been linked to skin cancer. Without light, however, there is no vitamin D produced and the patient may become ill physically or mentally. A moderate amount of light is necessary for skin and body health (WHO, 2013).

Personal Cleanliness

In all areas of patient care, a clean and safe home and personal environment support health, prevent illness, and preserve skin integrity. If a patient's home or living environment is not clean, if the skin is exposed to noxious factors such as urine or feces, or if the patient is exposed to a dirty environment due to poor ventilation, illness and skin breakdown can occur. Additionally, a patient who is left immobile in any environment without clean clothing and bed linens may be the victim of neglect. This situation demands immediate intervention. If education of the patient, family members, or caregivers does not produce results, outside authorities such as the Bureau for the Aging must be notified (Agency for Healthcare Research and Quality [AHRQ], 2008). If the patient is in immediate danger, call 911 or the local police. You can call the Elder Abuse Hotline or contact the Elder Abuse Agency in your state (see Appendix I).

Ensuring that a person is clean and dry has a dramatic effect on the skin. Experts agree the three most important steps to skin care are gentle washing, prevention of moisture-related damage, and the use of barrier and emolliating creams on a consistent basis (AHRQ, n.d.).

SKIN ASSESSMENT

The use of a pressure ulcer risk assessment tool is only the first step in assessing a patient's health status. A thorough skin assessment goes hand in hand with risk assessment. In order to successfully complete the assessment, the patient is observed from head to toe. Each part of the body is looked at, including the back of the head, ears, nose bridge, back, buttocks, sacrum, any abdominal folds, feet, heels, and ankles. Any part of the body may be exposed to pressure/friction or shear.

Case Study

An elderly woman came into an acute care facility with nose bleeds and clotting abnormalities. She routinely wore support hose. She was essentially immobile, sitting in a hard chair most of the day. When she was admitted to the emergency department, she refused to remove her

(continued)

Case Study *(continued)*

stockings so they were not removed. When she was admitted to the nursing unit, she agreed to have her stockings removed for a skin assessment. When the stockings were removed, the patient had large, plate-size hematomas on each calf, essentially caused by sitting in the same position for long periods of time without movement to relieve the pressure. Though the ulcers were most likely due to her bleeding abnormality, they would have been noted much earlier if her clothing were completely removed. She required emergency surgery to open each site to relieve the pressure and prevent further damage to her extremities. She had a long hospital stay and was eventually discharged to a rehabilitation facility.

FAST FACTS in a NUTSHELL

Remove all clothing to enable thorough skin assessment. The patient and family may need to be educated about the need to remove clothing to complete a thorough skin assessment.

This case study has implications for all nurses in all settings. It also has clear implications for home care but may present a challenge. Nurses in the home may see their patients infrequently, which makes a complete and thorough skin assessment even more important. If a patient is essentially immobile, frail, or has poor nutrition, it is important that the skin is assessed on a regular and frequent basis. How can this be accomplished? All encounters should be utilized for skin assessment. Others, such as family members or caregivers, may need to be initiated and educated to report findings. Nursing assistants should be empowered and educated to report abnormal findings.

Even if what was found is minor, larger issues could be prevented (AHRQ, n.d.).

A thorough skin assessment is actually a process. The entire body is examined for abnormalities. The documentation of the initial assessment provides the basis for all other encounters. When the initial picture of the body is painted, others who are caring for the individual can readily know what is not normal. The process is completed by educating the patient about what you are doing, ensuring his or her comfort, and observing and touching the skin from head to toe (AHRQ, 2008).

When conducting a skin assessment for the first time, a health history helps in understanding findings. A health history begins with an organized interview with the patient and includes general health and state of wellness, family health history, physical limitations, psychosocial and spiritual health, and any history of skin conditions. Collecting this information can be accomplished through patient interview, chart review, and from family members. Include information about the family history, particularly if the patient is living in an extended family environment. Be careful to include details related to current medications and medication regimen, the patient's bathing and skin care routines, specific allergies and allergens (if known), and any problems caused by topical medications or skin care products. Be meticulous about documenting findings of the patient's health history.

Medications often affect the skin and wound healing. It is important to understand exactly what medications the patient is taking. There are medications that actually impede healing. Common medications that affect healing include corticosteroids, nonsteroidal anti-inflammatory drugs (NSAIDs), antibiotics, chemotherapy, nicotine, anticoagulants, immunosuppressive drugs such as drugs for rheumatoid arthritis, and vasoconstrictors. It is also important to know if the patient takes any over-the-counter or herbal medications that may have some of these properties.

The skin provides a first-line defense against invasion of a variety of infectious organisms. It also reflects general body health, and so, careful inspection of this important organ provides critical clues as to possible problems lurking underneath the skin. Various aspects of skin assessment include observing for:

- Skin temperature
- Dryness
- Changes in skin texture
- Bruising
- Itching
- Changes in nail composition, which may indicate malnutrition or other malady of the nail
- Appearance of skin; it should have uniform appearance, thickness, and symmetry
- Integrity of skin; note lesions, cracks, fissures, ulcers, or any other alteration

Skin Assessment Techniques

1. Inspection = Purposeful Observation
Skin is normally smooth and moist with the same general skin tone. Check the patient's skin from head to toe. Findings can include:

- Pallor in the oral mucosa or in the conjunctiva of the eyes
- Cyanosis in the nail beds, nose extremities
- Jaundice in the sclera of the eyes or palms
- Hyperpigmentation from variation in melanin deposits or blood flow
- Hypopigmentation, which may indicate vascular changes
- Scars or bruising
- Discoloration such as redness (erythema)

- Check nails for normal shape and contour
- Check if there is lack of or excessive hair and the health of hair

2. Palpation = lightly "touching" or applying pressure
   When the skin is palpated, findings can reveal:

- Moisture such as perspiration or incontinence
- Edema of extremities or sacrum
- Tenderness or painful to touch
- Turgor or if the skin is pliable
- Texture of the skin, such as dry patches or psoriasis

3. Smell—olfaction
   Use the sense of smell to indicate patient problems related to:

- Body odor
- Presence or absence of pungent odor
- Incontinence
- Odor related to infection or the presence of bacteria
- Poor hygiene

Document, report, and implement treatment based on assessment findings (Hess, 2008). Frequent and consistent skin assessment will ensure early identification of skin breakdown at a stage that is responsive to early interventions (AHRQ, 2008). Skin assessment should be a standardized process not only in frequency but how it is done and what is included. Standardized skin assessment forms, whether electronic or written, will help all caregivers to be aware of exactly what is going on with the patient. Through this assessment a plan of care can be developed. The assessment indicates what is necessary in order to care for the patient (AHRQ, 2008).

There are barriers to doing a thorough skin assessment. Staff may not feel there is adequate time to do a complete assessment given their current workload. However, this is part of the initial patient assessment and regular patient care, and it allows for care to be determined. The skin assessment process is mandatory and focused but should be simple and without burden so that it is done properly and regularly.

All levels of staff should feel comfortable to report abnormal findings. Nursing assistants and caregivers who are doing much of the basic care need to feel that what they see on the patient is important. Skin care education should be a regular part not only of orientation but continuing in order to maintain ongoing competency of care. Simple tools can also be developed (such as a body outline) where nursing assistants can document their findings. These tools should be used in all care discussions about the patient (AHRQ, 2012).

MANAGING PRESSURE POINTS

Pressure points are bony areas of the body where ulcers can occur due to the pressure on the skin covering the bone. These points include the ear, shoulder, elbow, hip, thigh, leg, and heel (Figure 4.1). When the body is positioned on these sites without pressure relief, an ulcer can quickly occur. As part of the skin assessment it is necessary to check skin at these sites. Each issue noted should be carefully documented. Protection of these areas is essential.

Pressure to any of the areas shown in Figure 4.1 can occur when least expected. If a patient is sitting in a chair inappropriately or for long periods, ulcers can occur at the coccyx or sacrum or even the backs of the calves or thighs. If a patient has the blanket too tight for a long period of time, the tops of the toes could develop an ulcer. Equipment can create ulcerations to the back of the ears or nose. All

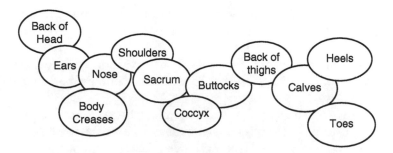

FIGURE 4.1 Key pressure points.

areas where there is likelihood that pressure can occur from within or from external sources need to be observed frequently for issues.

═══════════════════════════════*FAST FACTS in a NUTSHELL*

The sense of smell can provide indications about a patient's health status. Old dressings or unclean clothing often have an odor. If the odor permeates the room, however, this can indicate serious infection.

ASSESSING THE OBESE PATIENT

Assessing the skin of a bariatric surgery patient can be a challenge. Obese patients are prone to pressure ulcers. Changes in the skin can occur simply due to the skin-to-weight ratio and the decreased perfusion of fatty tissue. Bariatric patients often have pressure ulcers under the pannus (abdominal flap) and in other skin folds caused by the weight on delicate skin. The skin at these areas can have decreased blood supply and the skin may actually become necrotic. Because these areas are moist, they are especially prone to infection and poor healing.

Bariatric patients are prone to a variety of skin conditions. Not only are their tissues affected but they also often have a deficit of self-care resulting in poor hygiene and skin breakdown. Morbidly obese patients often have poor circulation and can develop ulcerations of the extremities. Though not necessarily from pressure, these ulcers can weep large amounts of fluid from the amount of edema in the underlying tissues. The moisture may need to be controlled with dressings to collect the drainage. It is important to keep the pressure off of these sites through positioning and elevation (Muir, 2009).

It is important to inspect the skin under the pannus, between the thighs, in the groin areas, and the posterior aspects of the legs on a frequent and regular basis. Unusual creases may exist on bariatric patients, such as at the base of the head; these creases warrant careful observation. Equipment such as lifts and pulls should be used carefully and readily to avoid further injury to the patient or to the caregiver. Bariatric equipment is specialized and requires education and training (Rush, 2009).

The number of patients who are morbidly obese has dramatically increased over the past decade. It is described as one of the world's most prominent health problem. According to WHO (2013), more than 300 billion adults are considered overweight, and 1 million are morbidly obese. Nurses seek to provide respectful care while protecting their own health and well-being (WHO, 2013).

The science of bariatrics is aimed at providing health care for those who are extremely obese. The most common method used to determine if a patient is overweight is the determination of his or her body mass index (BMI). Obese patients will have a BMI of greater than 30 while those who are severely obese will have a BMI of greater than 40

(WHO, 2013). Standard practice has been to initiate the use of bariatric equipment (Table 4.1) in patients who are greater than 350 pounds. This weight exceeds that recommended by standard equipment.

Immobility of obese patients puts them at high risk for pressure ulcer development. Mobility presents a challenge for the obese patient and this challenge increases with age. It is important to protect delicate skin while providing the safest possible care. Devices that are weight appropriate are the first step. Prior to or on admission, it is important to determine the equipment needed to safely care for the obese patient. Without the proper equipment, the facility should not accept the patient because the facility is not meeting the standard of care for the obese patient.

Transferring the bariatric patient can be risky for the patient and caregiver. There are multiple steps to the process and several considerations when using bariatric equipment, especially patient lifts. First, the equipment must be appropriate for the weight of the patient. This is dictated by the manufacturer. Equipment weight limits should be clearly displayed. Second, the process for use must be clear and spelled out for all who use it (a diagram is easy for all caregivers to follow). Third, everyone that uses the equipment must be educated on its use with periodic follow-up and review.

FAST FACTS in a NUTSHELL

Prior to a patient's admission, the patient's needs for equipment must be spelled out, especially when related to weight and what the patient will need to function safely. Using this method, safety for the patient and caregiver can be ensured.

TABLE 4.1 Bariatric Equipment Available to Provide Safe Patient Care

Personal Equipment	Prevention Equipment	Lifts
Walkers, canes	Bariatric low air loss mattresses/beds (Examples: Medline, Invacare, Drive, Lumex, ArjoHuntleigh)	Sit-to-stand lifts (Examples: Vanderlift, Hoyer, Stand-Aid, Sara Lift, Stella Lift, Stand Assist Lift, Sit-to-Stand, and Stand-Up Lifts)
Wheelchairs	Bariatric pressure relief cushions (Examples: Barifoam, EHOB, Gel Supreme, Posy, Trifor, ArjoHuntleigh)	Sling lifts (slings are designed for lift to chair or lift to toilet/commode) (Examples: Invacare, Lumex, Apex, Hoyer)
Regular bariatric bed or hospital beds	Protective dressings in larger sizes (Examples: Mölnlycke Mepilex, Smith & Nephew Allevyn, Convatec Aquacel Foam, Coloplast Biatain)	Patient slide assists (Examples: Apex Bariatric Turner, HoverMatt)
Scooters	Bariatric heel protectors and boots (Examples: Skil-Care, Prevalon, EHOB, AliMed DM Systems heel lifts)	Ceiling lifts (Examples: Hoyer, Traxx system, Voyager, Liko)
Commodes	Bariatric chairs and recliners	
Personal recliners	Wheelchairs for use in facility	
Safety bars equipped to handle patients over 300 pounds		

Source: Vieria (2008).

OUTPATIENTS AND PRESSURE ULCERS

Patients who are receiving routine treatment such as chemotherapy, fluids, or blood are actually at high risk for pressure ulcer development. Pressure ulcer prevention in this type of patient is often ignored. They are usually sitting for long periods—often over 2 hours—and may be prone to infection. Pressure ulcers develop due to long periods of immobility. In addition the prescribed medication may cause diarrhea. Skin assessment typically does not include pressure points such as the sacrum or coccyx.

Nurses who care for patients in outpatient treatment facilities need to be aware of pressure ulcer potential in their patients. Prevention tools such as chair cushions help in this type of setting. Patients can even be instructed to bring their cushion with them when they come back for treatment. Patients may need to be instructed to shift weight frequently, use a chair cushion if they are going to be sitting for any length of time, and to check the buttocks and gluteal cleft for ulcers or alteration in skin integrity. Caregivers and patients need to be made partners in care and to report any changes in the skin.

═══════════════════════════*FAST FACTS in a NUTSHELL*

Pay attention to the patient. Because a patient is able to ambulate and is released home, the skin may be ignored. If the patient is sitting for a period of time and has health issues or comorbidities, the patient and caregivers need instructions about pressure relief. Education about what to report could also prevent skin breakdown.

Once the patient's risk is determined and the skin is thoroughly assessed, it is up to the caregiver to prevent pressure ulcers from occurring. Because of the cost and patient harm associated with pressure ulcers, prevention is essential. Care is needed to ensure a pressure ulcer does not occur or does not progress. The next chapter will focus on prevention.

Preventing Pressure Ulcers

5

Pressure Ulcer Prevention

It has already been established that pressure ulcers cause patient harm. They are associated with adverse health effects, poor social well-being and interaction, high treatment costs, and overall detriment to quality of life. Preventing pressure ulcers in any setting is linked to the quality of care provided in that venue. Chronic ulcers can take a long time to heal and treatment can be costly. It is therefore better to prevent the ulcers from occurring in the first place (Hess, 2009).

Upon completion of this chapter, the reader will be able to:

1. Identify two techniques that can be utilized to prevent pressure ulcers
2. Discuss the basics of effective skin care
3. Define what is meant by moisture-associated skin damage

PREVENTION METHODOLOGY

The pressure ulcer risk assessment tool used in a particular facility should dictate the care provided to the individual patient. The Joint Commission, which surveys an organization's compliance with specific standards, and the Centers for Medicare and Medicaid Services (CMS), which focuses on organizations meeting specific regulations, both require that there is an individualized plan of care. This is evident in all health care settings. Nurses need to articulate the plan of care for the patient, which should be individualized, include a multidisciplinary team, and prioritize patient needs. Nursing interventions are based on findings from the patient assessment (Vanderbilt, 2012).

Based on use of the Braden Risk Assessment Tool, there are prevention tools that can be linked to the individual score. The interventions are based on the following findings and care is planned accordingly:

Braden score of 15 to 18—Low risk

a. Frequent repositioning and turning
b. Encourage patient to reposition self if able
c. Ensure that patient's activity and mobility are maximized
d. Protect heels
e. Use pressure-reducing surfaces

Braden score of 13 to 14—Moderate risk

a. Use above methods but include routine repositioning
b. Use bolsters or wedges to maintain position if needed

Braden score of 10 to 12—High risk

a. Increase turning frequency
b. Do small shifts of position especially for those patients who are very debilitated or critical

c. Consider pressure-relieving surfaces for bed and in chair
d. Manage moisture, nutrition, and friction/shear

Braden score of 9 or below—Very high risk

a. Use above interventions
b. Use pressure-relieving surface when in bed and in chair (Ayello, 2012)

These prevention tools based on the Braden Scale for Predicting Pressure Sore Risk are effective in pressure ulcer prevention and will be discussed in more detail in upcoming sections.

POSITIONING

Frequent and consistent repositioning is important in decreasing pressure, friction, and shear. This is a common nursing tool and has been used for many years; however, it may not always be utilized effectively. The usual rule for changes in patient repositioning is every 2 hours. This rule can be linked to the point when damage to skin occurs. Patients who are very ill may actually require more frequent repositioning as their skin is very frail. Nurses may not be appropriately repositioning patients as some studies indicate that nurses cannot meet positioning requirements due to staffing and workload (Lyder, 2008).

A regimen that alters patient position every 2 hours is a good starting point. Frequent skin assessment can determine if the frequency of repositioning is adequate for a particular patient. If there is no erythema over bony prominences after the repositioning period, then the frequency is sufficient for that patient. The amount of repositioning also depends on the individual patient. Sometimes subtle shifts are all that can be done with a critically ill patient but that off-loading of pressure is important to maintaining skin integrity. Therefore, positioning, like all types of nursing care, is individualized (Wounds International [International Review], 2010).

It is best if patients reposition themselves but patients may not understand the implications of repositioning. Education for patients, families, and caregivers only increases prevention efforts (Agency for Healthcare Research and Quality [AHRQ], 2008). Patients who are in pain may not reposition themselves. Patients who are young or relatively healthy may appear able to reposition themselves but may not do so because it hurts too much. If patients do not reposition themselves and are found in the same position frequently, they need help in understanding the importance of repositioning themselves or must be offered help to reposition. Nursing interventions aimed at pain management can go a long way in preventing skin issues (Wound Ostomy and Continence Nurses Society [WOCN], 2010).

Proper positioning of patients to prevent pressure ulcers is accomplished by:

- Repositioning a patient on alternate sides at least every 2 hours
- Protecting pressure points and delicate skin when changing a patient's position
- Positioning to ensure that body parts are not touching or rubbing against each other
- Using sufficient tools for the patient to maintain the position—for example, pillows or bolsters

Propping a patient to maintain an alternate position can be accomplished by use of pillows, soft towels, or blankets. Soft foam props are available and, though they may be expensive, are a better alternative as the shapes help accomplish the best positioning possible. Carefully check the patient after positioning to ensure that body parts are not rubbing or that one part is not causing pressure to another. Reposition chairbound or wheelchair-bound clients every hour. In addition, if the client is capable, have him or her do small weight shifts every 15 minutes.

FAST FACTS in a NUTSHELL

A side-lying person may need pillows or soft padding between legs, feet, and ankles or even under folds of the pannus. Other body parts that may require protection include hands (if the patient's fingers are clenched) and the tip of the ears. Soft washcloths are a good padding source.

Protecting Heels

Preventing heel ulcers can present a challenge. Patients develop heel ulcers based on the risk factors already identified but they may also occur due to peripheral vascular disease, diabetes, hip fractures, obesity, or post major surgery. Heels that are compromised often appear soft, pink, and nonblanchable (i.e., not able to return to original circulatory state), or blistered. These ulcers can be devastating as they can affect a person's mobility. Heels are a pressure point and the skin is soft and moves easily. Friction from rubbing while in bed is also common (Swezy, 2011). Protecting patients through positioning and heel protection are simple methods to prevent skin breakdown.

Heels are protected by lifting them off of the surface.

- Short-term support: Pillows can be used especially in acute care or in the home. Pillows are placed lengthwise behind the knee to the heel to elevate the heel (National Pressure Ulcer Advisory Panel, 2009; WOCN, 2010).
- Long-term prevention: There are many products that produce heel protection in the form of a soft plastic or cloth boot. When using these products, ensure they fit the patient well and that they do produce the result of keeping the heels off of the surface. Follow manufacturers' recommendations; some patients may need a sock or padding to prevent friction.

====================================*FAST FACTS in a NUTSHELL*

If using a pressure-relieving boot, make sure it is appropriate for the patient's weight. Boots may not be appropriate for patients who are edematous as they may actually cause damage through constriction. Check the appropriate weight limit as well. A larger patient may need a bariatric boot.

PROPER LIFTING TECHNIQUES

Appropriate patient lifting is another way to prevent pressure ulcers. Lift patients up and off of a surface; never drag from side to side. This may be easier said than done especially when patients are very large or stiff. Nurses, however, need to think defensively. If the patient is difficult to move because he or she is stiff or large, then pulling is not the answer. Using lift sheets, easy movers, or patient lifts is the answer. If the patient is dragged against the surface, this can result in skin damage from friction and shear (Hess, 2009).

Lifting patients can present a challenge. It is also a common way that staff members get hurt. Patient lifts are used whenever possible to protect both the patient and the caregiver. There are standing lifts, sling lifts, or ceiling lifts as well as smooth movers, Hover mats, or slip sheets. When positioning a patient, use common sense. Use draw sheets and incontinence pads in combination with a log roll or moving the patient from side to side.

Safe practices:

- Adjust beds or other surfaces to waist height and as close to you as possible.
- Lower the rails on the bed or stretcher, working on the side closest to the individual.

- Equipment and treatment items should be close at hand when working to avoid the caregiver having to stretch to reach the items.
- Assess a patient's level of mobility before lifting or moving.
- Use safe handling techniques with all patients and do not move someone yourself unless you know the patient's abilities.

Just as nursing assistants and caregivers are empowered to report abnormal findings in patients' skin, they should also be educated to report unsafe practices in patient care routines. Facilities need to provide training to all involved so that issues with patient care and transfers are easily identified. This too is an important part of ongoing competency to minimize risk and injury, not only to staff members but also to the patients (Occupational Safety and Health Administration [OSHA], 2009).

MOISTURE-WICKING PADS

When a patient is incontinent it is common practice to apply incontinence briefs. Patients may actually request to wear briefs to avoid soiling or wetting. All diapers or briefs increase moisture because they are occlusive and trap moisture between the diaper and the skin. Warmth is produced and when combined with moisture and ammonia, skin breakdown can occur. Some briefs are so absorbent that it may be difficult to tell if they are wet. When used for fecal incontinence, acid is trapped against the skin.

Many health care facilities have moved away from using briefs except when a patient is ambulating. Moisture is decreased using underpads that wick and hold fluid away from the skin. Moisture-wicking pads do not trap heat and moisture next to the body, and it can readily be seen when they need to be changed. The cost of these products may make some facilities shy away from using them; however, when compared to the cost of a pressure ulcer, the use is well worth the expense. A lift sheet may be needed when using underpads. Examples include Covidien, Medline, and Attends. Avoid pads with plastic on the outside or as an inner lining. These pads hold moisture and can actually cause moisture-related skin issues (Hess, 2009).

═════════════════════════════════**FAST FACTS in a NUTSHELL**

Include moisture-wicking pads for use on most patients. They help patients' skin stay dry. Because they are more expensive than the reusable pads, one pad is sufficient. Bariatric products are also available.

PREVENTING FRICTION AND SHEAR

Friction and shear have been discussed briefly in the beginning chapters. However, they are key concepts for preventing pressure ulcers. Friction is the force that occurs from rubbing two surfaces together. Shear is a result of gravity pushing down on the body toward something that is resistant such as the bed or chair. When friction and shear are combined, the results can be devastating. The body moves, but the skin or surface does not. Friction can cause minor to substantial skin impairment. Friction alone does not directly cause a pressure ulcer and not all friction injuries are pressure ulcers. For example, as a result of skin rubbing against a sheet, an abrasion can develop. However, friction can contribute to shear strain in the tissue; add pressure from inside or outside and a pressure ulcer can occur (Antokal, 2012).

Knowing this, it is important to prevent the combined forces of friction and shear (Table 5.1).

TABLE 5.1 Causes of Friction and Shear

Causes	Remedies
Head of bed elevated without clinical correlation	• Ensure head of bed is elevated only for clinical reasons or for meals • Patient rounds done after meals should include ensuring that the patient's head is not elevated greater than 30 degrees (unless it is clinically necessary)
Restless patient	• Use soft socks when a patient is in bed • Ensure that antiembolism stockings are the correct size • Use no-sting barrier cream as protection • Heel protectors • Soft sheepskin or bath blanket at bottom of bed to prevent patient from rubbing feet against sheet
Inappropriate patient lifts	• Caregivers should be educated to move patients using a lift sheet • Lift patients off of the bed instead of dragging • Ensure caregivers have sufficient help to move the patient • Ask the patient to assist if possible
Pulling a pad or brief out from under a patient	• Place pads between legs instead of under if possible • Avoid adult diapers when in bed • Turn patient to remove soiled clothing • Instruct all caregivers that pulling pads or briefs from under a patient can result in skin injury
Improperly assisting patient out of bed or without proper support	• Two people should always be available to avoid falls
Dry skin	• Avoid hot water • Use emollients (list of emollients and moisturizers discussed elsewhere) • Ensure patient's skin is not moist from perspiration or incontinence

(continued)

TABLE 5.1 Causes of Friction and Shear (*continued*)	
Causes	**Remedies**
Patients that sag or slide in chair	• Assist patient to stand and reposition him or her in the chair • Lift and reposition the patient using patient lift or at least two caregivers • Use positioning cushions or bolsters to ensure patient does not slide • If patient is in a wheelchair, use a chair cushion that relieves pressure
Patient transfers using poor technique	• When using a sliding board to transfer a patient, inspect the skin carefully for friction • A trapeze may help the patient move quicker • Use a patient lift if the sliding board is causing skin injury

Source: Nurse Leader Insider, 2009; Wounds International [International Review], 2010.

SUPPORT SURFACES

Support surfaces are an integral part of pressure ulcer prevention programs. Product selection can be tedious but the ultimate goal is to provide the best care for the patient at the least cost. These surfaces are used based on the patient's skin status. Surfaces can be pressure reducing or pressure relieving. Pressure reduction is important but these surfaces do not provide the prevention capacity of the pressure-relieving surface. Pressure-relieving surfaces allow for patients to be positioned without the mattress bottoming out against the bed surface causing pressure to individual body parts.

There are pressure-relieving products for standard bed mattresses as well as specialty beds. They are also available for operating room tables and stretchers. Static beds and/or mattresses that do not require a power source and redistribute localized pressure. Dynamic beds or mattresses use a power source to alternate currents in order to redistribute pressure.

Because the choice can be difficult, specialty beds and mattresses will be discussed in more detail in upcoming chapters.

There are also pressure-relieving cushions for chairs. Remember, patients that are out of bed for prolonged periods of time may develop pressure ulcers. It is necessary to shift a patient's position, especially if sitting on a hard surface. Pressure-relieving cushions can be air, gel, foam, or mixed gel and foam. Manufacturers that produce specialty beds often also produce chair cushions; therefore, cushions will be included in the discussion of specialty beds.

FAST FACTS in a NUTSHELL

If pressure-relieving products such as mattresses or cushions are utilized, ensure that they are readily accessible. Avoiding delay can be very important, especially for the frailest patients or those that have serious ulcers.

BASIC SKIN CARE TOOLS

Cleansing

Gentle daily skin cleansing is essential not only for health but to prevent skin issues. Using strong soaps actually emulsifies the lipids in the skin and increases the pH of the skin mantle. The skin is slightly acidic so raising the pH decreases the natural skin barrier, which can lead to skin damage. The key is to use gentle cleansers for routine care and to remove feces or urine (Table 5.2). In addition, care should be taken not to rub the skin, which may cause friction injuries for patients with frail skin, such as the ill or elderly. Routine care is done as gently as possible to avoid skin damage. Education may be necessary to frontline caregivers to ensure this is the case.

Some basic skin care rules include:

- Assess skin regularly—use skin care as a method for skin observation
- Clean skin at time of soiling; urine and feces can be acidic and can remove the natural skin barrier
- Avoid hot water and irritating cleaning agents that may dry the skin and leave it open to injury. Bathe or shower in warm water
- Do not rub skin vigorously or massage skin over bony prominences; do not dry or cleanse vigorously
- Limit bathing time to 5 minutes per shower or bath
- Humidify the external environment in the winter or year round if the climate is dry or air in the facility/home is dry
- Use gentle cleansers as opposed to soap

Skin is cleansed using mild detergents. These mild cleansers will not remove the protective mantle, do not dry the skin, and provide moisture to the skin. Some facilities require the use of antibacterial soaps or washes. These are appropriate within acute care or long-term care facilities; however, these may cause dryness or irritation. Some patients may have skin eruption from these products. Plain warm water (not hot) is just as effective for cleansing, especially for dry or sensitive skin, and may be necessary if a patient's skin is scaly or inflamed (Ayello, 2012).

There are many skin care products on the market and again the choice can be confusing. When choosing a cleanser, ensure it is gentle and adds moisture rather then removes it. There are two general rules for skin cleansers for patients:

- Gentle cleansers remove dirt and provide moisture
- Cleansers with surfactant assist in gently removing feces or urine without vigorous rubbing

TABLE 5.2 Cleansers		
Type of Cleanser	**Use**	**Examples**
Foam	Most are total body cleansers. Some are rinsed off; some can remain on skin	Convatec Aloe Vesta cleansing foam, DermaRite Renew, DermaRad Relief, Tea Tree Foam cleanser, Remedy cleansing foam, Coloplast Sproam body wash
Liquid/body wash	Can be used on wash-cloths or in water. Generally pleasing for patients	Convatec Aloe Vesta skin cleanser or conditioner, Thera body wash, Secura personal cleanser, Coloplast bedside care skin cleanser/peri-wash
Spray	Easy to use especially for hard-to-reach places. Often no rubbing is needed	3M Cavilon spray cleanser, ProShield incontinent spray and cleanser, Remedy spray cleanser, Convatec Aloe Vesta spray cleanser
Wipes	Some are for peri-anal area and some are total body wash. Total body wash often adds moisture, eliminates extra washing steps	Prevail disposable washcloth, Sage Comfort care wipes, Chicopee soft patient wipes, Clinell patient wipes, Reynard patient wipes, Medline soft wipes

Source: Ayello, 2012; Gray, 2011.

===*FAST FACTS in a NUTSHELL*

Assess patient's skin after cleansing. It should appear moist and supple, not dry and parched. If this occurs, the cleanser is too strong for the individual.

Humidification of the Environment

It has already been discussed that humidified air prevents dry skin. Humidification provides moist air and a moist environment for the skin. When the air inside is dry it removes moisture from the body. Dry skin is not protected and injury can occur. It is therefore necessary to put water back into the air through humidification. Humidifiers can be as simple as a vaporizer or as complicated as a whole air purifying system. A facility may have single humidifiers or may actually have air filter systems. In the home it may be necessary to ensure the humidifier being used is safe and clean.

Humidifiers can be fairly inexpensive. Most run on water in a tank that is filled regularly. Humidification can actually moisturize skin and lips. Cool mist can also relieve dry nasal passages and ease congestion by liquefying secretions. Skin in a humidified environment is moist, maintaining protection for the rest of the body (Warner, 2009).

Use of Emollients and Moisturizers

The use of emollients and moisturizers during skin care can also prevent friction. Moisturizers can ease cracked skin and provide comfort. The use of gentle barrier creams is an essential part of a skin care program (Lyder, 2008). These creams ease friction and protect the skin from incontinence and other types of moisture. Nurses and facilities would be wise to have these creams readily available. All involved in patient care should be educated to use them liberally on a regular basis. Moisturizing patient's skin and providing barriers against assault from urine and feces is one of the first lines of defense against pressure ulcers.

The mechanism of action of moisturizers involves the stratum corneum layer of the skin. Moisture initiates in the epidermis, works its way up to the surface, and is lost by evaporation. The stratum corneum is an active membrane. If the skin is flattened because of age or with loss of cholesterol and fatty acids, the water barrier function is damaged. There is no water to be utilized because it is not there. Dry skin occurs when the moisture content of the skin is less than 10% and there is a loss of continuity of the stratum corneum or active membrane (Wounds International [International Review], 2010).

Functions of moisturizing skin include:

- Repairs skin barrier
- Increases the water content while reducing water loss
- Restores the lipid barrier's ability to attract, hold, and move water through the body
- Moisturizers hydrate the stratum corneum and reduce water loss
- Emollients make skin supple
- Act as the skin's own barrier

Moisturizers should soak into the skin while barriers or emollients stay on the skin as protection (Table 5.3). Humectants in moisturizers attract water when applied and actually draw water away from the skin. If water is evaporated from the skin, then dryness can actually increase. Humectants in moisturizers are best avoided. These include glycerin, sorbitol, urea, alpha hydroxyl acids (i.e., lactic acid), and other sugars (DermNet NZ, 2012).

Moisture-Associated Skin Damage (MASD)

The concept of moisture is different from the skin being moisturized—this can be confusing. Moisture that is toxic such as from bowel, bladder, or stomach contents can irritate the

TABLE 5.3 Moisturizers

Types of Moisturizing Products	Use	Examples
Lotions	Provide moisture to skin, soak in easily. Skin becomes supple with improved elasticity after use	Eucerin, Lubriderm, Keri-Lotion, 3M Cavilon moisture lotion, Convatec Aloe Vesta lotion, Coloplast Sween lotion
Creams	Thicker but with the same advantage as lotion. May provide healing abilities for patients with dry skin related to vascular issues	Eucerin, Calmoseptine cream, Medseptic protectant cream, Coloplast Sween cream, Convatec Sensi-care moisturizing body cream
Barrier creams	Protect skin from the assault of acid such as feces or urine. Stays on skin; should be able to visualize cream but should remove easily	Convatec Aloe Vesta barrier cream, Calmoseptine ointment, Coloplast anti-fungal barrier cream, Smith & Nephew, Secura protectant
Barrier wipes/liquid	Protect skin by providing a thin barrier. Stays on skin but not necessarily to moisturize, protective in nature	Coloplast Prep protective skin barrier, DermaRite StingFree prep pad, 3M Cavilon No Sting barrier, Convatec No Sting barrier film, Allkare protective barrier, Bard barrier film

Source: AHRQ (2008).

skin and cause damage. Moisturizing with emollients adds a barrier to the skin and prevents dryness and cracking as well as preventing toxic moisture from affecting the skin. MASD is caused by long-term exposure to moisture attributed to urine, stool, wound drainage, perspiration, saliva, and stomach contents. Ulcers occur when moisture is not controlled and other factors are present such as pressure, friction, or shear. It is important to identify, treat, or block moisture from affecting the skin and to clearly identify what has caused the skin damage—is the damage a pressure ulcer?

The pH of the skin is slightly acidic, which provides protection from the assault of moisture, outside elements, and the suppression of coliform bacteria. Moisture from incontinence of urine and stool, perspiration, wound exudates, or effluent from an ostomy for prolonged periods can cause skin damage. Damage occurs because of the effects of excessive moisture over time that essentially remove the protective mantle of healthy skin (Gray, 2011).

There are four types of skin damage caused by excessive moisture:

1. *Incontinence-associated dermatitis*: Caused by stool or urine and characterized by erythema and inflammation of the skin, and erosion of the top layers of skin (denuded skin).
2. *Intertriginous dermatitis*: Caused by perspiration usually between skin folds or creases, resulting in skin becoming eroded, red, and inflamed.
3. *Peri-wound moisture-associated dermatitis*: Erythema and inflammation within 4 cm of a wound, resulting in erosion. The skin becomes denuded or damaged because of a combination of drainage and traumatic removal of adhesives.
4. *Peri-stomal moisture-associated dermatitis*: Erythema and inflammation on the skin around a stoma or erosion caused by exposure to urine under the skin barrier of the ostomy appliance.

It is well known that inflamed, excoriated, or damaged skin is prone to infection. Although infections vary, there is no mistaking that moisture-related damage removes the protective mantle, leaving delicate skin exposed to further assault (Gray, 2011).

Body folds and creases are especially prone to rashes and infection. Body folds are typically higher temperature than skin that is exposed to light and air. Another factor contributing to the creation of an environment conducive to the development of rashes and infection is that moisture and perspiration become trapped within the skin fold. Some common examples are:

* Fungal rashes
* Intertrigo rashes

Intertrigo refers to a rash within a body fold that is characterized by red, raw skin often with satellite lesions. This is particularly common in people who are obese, because of the high temperature and trapped moisture within the skin folds. These rashes are worsened by friction between the skin folds. The moist environment actually supports overgrowth of the bacteria and yeasts that are normal skin flora (DermNet NZ, 2012).

The common denominator among the different types of MASD is that the moisture is toxic or cannot evaporate. Keeping skin clean, dry, and *moisturized* is a primary goal in prevention and treatment of MASD as well as other skin issues. Most skin eruptions are caused by yeast, most often *Candida*. This rash appears red, raw, and pimply with lesions that satellite from the main source.

Interventions to prevent and treat MASD:

* Remove irritants from the skin as quickly as possible
* Apply barrier creams liberally and frequently to susceptible skin areas
* Use moisture-wicking underpads especially with patients who are frequently moist
* Avoid use of adult diapers that do not wick moisture (underpads can actually be placed between the legs and underneath the buttocks to wick this moisture)
* Control moisture in body creases—there are fabric products formulated to wick moisture in these areas and some have silver (antibacterial) properties
* Use antifungal creams or powders on areas that are affected by these types of rashes (Table 5.4)

- Use mattresses or overlays that create a microclimate to eliminate moisture. Moisture-wicking mattresses/sheets draw air down through the mattress cover along with heat moisture and odors (Gray, 2011).

Some of these interventions are expensive and the facility/agency should choose what is appropriate for its patients. What is important to remember is that keeping skin clean and dry goes a long way to prevent skin breakdown.

TABLE 5.4 Antifungal/Intertrigo Treatment

Treatment	Properties	Examples
Topical antifungal creams	Usually two times daily. Skin should be as dry as possible when applying. Apply slightly around perimeter of rash.	Clotrimazole (Lotrimin), Nystatin (Mycostatin), Tinactin
Topical antifungal creams with steroid	Patients who have severe rash and can tolerate steroid application	Clotrimazole, Betamethazone, Nystatin/ Triamcinolone (Mycolog)
Oral antifungal	Used when infection is intensive or severe and resists topical treatment	Fluconazole (Diflucan), Ketoconazole (Nizoral tablets)
Other remedies	Adjunct therapy used along with topical or oral products or if these products are contraindicated	Barrier creams such as Aloe Vesta antifungal cream; Terrasil pain and anti-itch cream; cloths to place into folds: Coloplast Interdry. At home, patients can actually dry skin with a fan or cool hair dryer to avoid irritaton

Source: Provider Synergis LLC (2010).

FAST FACTS in a NUTSHELL

Think defensively when doing patient care to prevent skin issue injury. Nurses in any setting can think about each patient encounter. Planning care allows nurses and all who provide patient care to ensure every step of care is effective and safe—assessment, routine care, treatment, and patient follow-up.

6

Nutrition and Pressure Ulcers

Nutrition is another consideration in the prevention and treatment of skin ulcers. Poor patient outcomes in general are a result of poor nutrition. The incidence of pressure ulcers increases when patients have significant weight loss or problems eating. Pressure ulcers also increase in patients who have poor nutrition, protein deficits, and dehydration. Without appropriate nutrients or a means to obtain them, organs are not fed and can cease to function.

Upon completion of this chapter, the reader will be able to:

1. Define what is meant by malnutrition
2. Discuss the importance of nutrition to skin
3. Identify two laboratory studies that can be used to indicate patients' nutritional status

ASSESSING NUTRITIONAL STATUS

Malnutrition refers to any imbalance in nutrition—undernutrition or overnutrition in the obese person. Malnutrition causes many health issues especially in the person with illness or comorbid conditions. Some of the effects include suppression of the immune system, muscle wasting, decreased wound healing, longer lengths of stay, and death. People who are hospitalized often have a combination of cachexia (severe loss of body weight, fat, and muscle due to increased protein catabolism) and malnutrition (Barker, 2011). Undernutrition, which refers to energy and protein deficits that can be reversed by providing appropriate nutrients, is more common (Little, 2013).

Nutrition is a fundamental aspect of patient care. It is a common deficit in patients who are ill, hospitalized, or in long-term care facilities. More than 85% of patients in long-term care have been reported to have nutrition deficits and over 40% of hospitalized patients are malnourished. The most serious type of malnutrition is protein-energy malnutrition. In this patient population there is a decreased absorption of protein and decreased energy. Protein is essential for cell production and to maintain homeostasis.

Risk assessment including nutrition status related to pressure ulcers has already been discussed. Nutrition status can be assessed using one of several available tools. The Mini-Nutritional Assessment and the Malnutrition Universal Screening tools are common but not used by all health care professionals. Use of the Braden Scale for Predicting Pressure Sore Risk assesses patients for nutrition deficits. This scale is used on admission, regularly, and with a change in patient condition. Once a deficit is found, clinical nutrition should be included in the care of the patient. If a patient is found to have an ulcer on admission to a facility, the team members should be consulted as soon as possible. The care of the patient with nutritional deficiency is best done by a multidisciplinary team (Dorner, 2009).

Patients that require multidisciplinary intervention:

- 5% or greater weight loss
- Refusal to eat or two meals a day where 50% or less is eaten
- No appetite

- Nausea or vomiting for 3 days or more
- Poor skin turgor, elasticity, or integrity
- Chronic infections, especially urinary tract infections
- Poor fluid intake

Wounds actually can cause malnutrition. Wounds cause hypermetabolic/catabolic states where the body is using more nutrients than are available. The breakdown of protein is required for all wound healing functions. Ulcers that are serious or are infected put more demands on the body systems. In addition, patients who are frail or elderly have a difficult time regaining or maintaining weight. It is therefore important to monitor not only intake but weight as well.

NUTRITIONAL MARKERS

There are several markers that can be used to determine if a patient has a nutritional deficit. Body measurements such as body mass index (BMI) or documentation of serial weights are used with patients. Checking a patient's skin integrity and elasticity at various body sites—such as the forearm and sacral area—can be a simple gauge of a patient's skin integrity. These checks are used to determine chronic undernutrition (Little, 2013).

Calculating a person's BMI is based on height and weight. BMI calculation:

- Underweight = less than 18.5
- Normal weight = 18.5 to 24.9
- Overweight = 25 to 29.9
- Obese = greater than 30

(Link to National Heart, Lung, and Blood Institute: www .nhlbi.nih.gov/guidelines/obesity/bmi_tbl.htm)

A nutrition assessment includes a biochemical analysis (Table 6.1). It must be noted that there is no one laboratory study that definitively determines a person's nutritional status. A person may appear ill or malnourished before the lab studies are noted. Albumin and pre-albumin can be an indicator but they are influenced by other factors such as hydration, extreme stress, or surgery (Little, 2013). It is more important to assess a patient's overall risk, as well as daily intake of fluids and food, changes in weight and skin integrity, overall health, and their medications (Dorner, 2009). A thorough assessment of nutrition status looks at the total patient.

═══════════════════════════════════════*FAST FACTS in a NUTSHELL*

Along with specific calculations such as how much the patient eats per meal or the patient's BMI, include general appearance, skin turgor, and elasticity in a nutrition assessment.

The goal of intervention in a patient's nutritional status is to promote health and healing. Energy (kilocalories) is provided through protein, carbohydrates, and fats. People with wounds have a higher energy requirement. Calories are calculated based on age, gender, weight, and activity. Calories are best attained through a healthy and balanced diet. Experts agree that diets should be somewhat liberal, allowing the person to have a broad food choice. The general rule is to provide 30 to 35 kilocalories per kilogram of body weight for people who have wounds, ulcers, or are under stress (Agency for Healthcare Research and Quality [AHRQ], 2008).

NUTRITIONAL REQUIREMENTS

• Patients need sufficient protein, which is responsible for cell multiplication, collagen, and connective tissue.

TABLE 6.1 Common Chemistry Studies to Assess Nutritional Status and Well-Being

Test	Reference Range (May Differ Slightly by Institution/Lab)	What Alteration Can Indicate
CBC	White cells: 5.0–10.0 × 10⁹/L; Red cells: 4.2–5.7 Hemoglobin: 13.2–16.9 Hematocrit: 38.5%–49%	These cells can be affected by malnutrition, which can decrease cell count
Complete metabolic panel	Glucose: 70–145 mg/dL Total protein: 6.8–4.3 Albumin: 3.4–5.4 Total calcium: 9.0–10.5 mg/dL BUN: 7–20 mg/dL Creatinine: 0.5–1.2 mg/dL Electrolytes: Sodium: 135–145 mEq/L Potassium: 3.5–5.0 Bicarbonate: 22–30 mmol/L Chloride: 98–108 mmol/L	Assesses kidney, electrolyte balance, acid–base balance, glucose, and blood protein. Can indicate malnutrition, dehydration
Serum iron	60 to 170 mcg/dL	Malnutrition and anemia
Serum magnesium	2.4–4.1 mg/dL	Malnutrition, diuretic use, chronic antacid use. Sometimes elevated when re-feeding, which needs to be monitored
Amylase	23–125 U/L	Chronic vomiting
Pre-albumin	12–50 mg/dL	Assesses nutrition status

Source: "Lab Studies On Line" (2013).

- Protein is necessary for healing at all phases. The usual requirement is 1.2 to 1.5 g per kg of body weight daily.
- Amino acids such as arginine and glutamine are also necessary as they are essential to build protein.

- Fluids may actually increase the oxygen in body tissues. Sufficient fluids must be given daily, being careful with patients who have fluid overload or renal problems.
- Micronutrients related to healing are usually obtained through a healthy diet. These are vitamin C (ascorbic acid), which works with iron; zinc, an antioxidant for collagen formation; and copper, which is needed for collagen cross-linking (Dorner, 2009; Little, 2013).

Stress increases the need for calories, protein, and hydration. Calories provide energy and are important for proper nutrition. Simply increasing calories may not be enough. Patients may not tolerate foods high in calories. Supplements may be necessary such as shakes, smoothies, and oral supplements.

Protein is important to sustain muscle mass, immune response, and skin integrity. Protein is in meat, fish, dairy, legumes, nuts, and seeds. High-protein diets are often intolerable. Supplements may include calories and protein. For protein requirements, it may be necessary to include powdered milk shakes, protein dense supplements, oral supplements, as well as shakes and smoothies.

Hydration is necessary for the body to function and to break down protein and calories. It is important to ensure that the patient has sufficient fluid intake. If the patient is unable to swallow thin liquids, thickened liquids may be necessary. A multidisciplinary team will need to decide on the appropriate intervention for each individual patient and that care is planned accordingly.

Supplementing a patient's nutrition can indeed be a challenge. Patients who cannot eat well or who have swallowing difficulties may need additional intervention. In general, providing a balanced, easy-to-eat diet that meets the person's food preferences is a good guide. Patients may need to be fed; this is often overlooked. It may be difficult to manage but patients need to be given sufficient time to be fed or to eat. Food may need to be warmed.

═══════════════════════════════════*FAST FACTS in a NUTSHELL*

If a patient is not going to be fed when trays are delivered, do not put the tray in the room. Think about a cold pureed meal sitting on the table for over an hour—appetizing? Or better yet, being hungry but unable to reach the tray or eat the food in front of you.

General rules when feeding a patient: Encourage the patient to fully consume the protein on the plate; document food likes and dislikes; encourage the patient to eat in an upright position; allow time for chewing; ensure the environment is clean and odor free; make sure the patient has teeth or dentures if offering foods that must be chewed; and offer fluids frequently (Hurd, n.d.).

Supplementing nutrition status can be done by thinking in a different manner. For example, patients drink liquids with their medications. Protocols that provide for liquid shakes or supplements to be given with medications accomplish multiple needs—patients get fluids, medications, as well as supplement. In addition, the clinical dietician may order Liquacel Protein supplement routinely. This provides liquid protein in small amounts. These protocols are a means by which some facilities ensure that their patients drink the supplements provided rather than have them sit on their bedside tables or in refrigerators.

Nutrition intervention again is multidisciplinary. Experts in nutrition are those who should provide for a person's nutrition goals. Caregivers and clinical dieticians work best together to meet patient needs. The following chapters will focus on additional methods to help patients maintain health, skin integrity, and promote healing.

7

Mobility and Pressure Ulcers

It has already been discussed that patient immobility is a major contributing factor in the development of pressure ulcers. Thus, increasing mobility for even the most critical patients can decrease the development of complications from immobility including pressure ulcers. Recent evidence has pointed to the development of a nurse-driven mobility protocol, which is being developed not only in acute and critical care situations, but also in the home and long-term care. Under specific guidelines, nurses are empowered to work with physical and occupational therapists to move the patient when they are safely ready to do so.

Multidisciplinary team goals for the patient are reviewed on a regular and consistent basis so that the patient's mobility goals can be met. In such cases it has been found that even patients in intensive care and those who are ventilated can be part of these protocols. Patient outcomes are positive with fewer complications from lack of mobility, medications such as vasopressors, and mechanical ventilation (Drolet, 2012).

Upon completion of this chapter, the reader will be able to:

1. Discuss the importance of increasing patient mobility not only to skin health but overall well-being
2. Identify two methods to increase patient mobility
3. Discuss patient mobility protocols as they relate to patient care

THE EFFECTS OF IMMOBILITY ON THE BODY

If patients are not mobilized, they become weak and lose essential functions. Increasing patients' mobility improves patient outcomes by preventing the consistent loss of muscle and body mass. Mobility is more than moving from one point to the next. Mobility assists patients to express emotions, meet basic needs, and perform activities of daily living. It enhances the body's ability to repair and heal. Bed rest, on the other hand, affects all body systems including the respiratory, cardiovascular, musculoskeletal, urinary and fecal elimination, integumentary and psychological systems.

If a patient is on bed rest, a patient's health status can quickly deteriorate. One week of bed rest can cause serious changes to the body:

1. Contractures can develop as skeletal muscles atrophy
2. Loss of muscle strength can be noted
3. Decreased volume of plasma circulation in the body, which causes stress on the cardiovascular system
4. Insulin resistance is developed
5. Visible weakness is noted, as well as a decrease in strength
6. Bones begin to deteriorate

In addition there is a decrease in lung capacity; an increased chance of deep vein thrombosis; loss of body mass; increased removal of calcium, nitrogen, and phosphorus from the body; decreased bone density; and decreased attention with altered behavior (King, 2012).

Immobility is also costly. Patients who are immobile because of illness only become more debilitated. They stay in critical care for longer periods. They must be hospitalized for longer periods and require increased rehabilitation. Because of this, acute care facilities are instituting early mobility programs not only for those who are on medical–surgical units but those in critical care units as well. We have already linked pressure ulcers to immobility, so with early mobilization the prevalence of pressure ulcers is also decreased.

Physiologically changing a patient's body position from lying to standing increases blood flow and heart rate, increases lung expansion, and improves oxygenation, which inevitably assists patients to heal. Psychologically both the patient and the family see progress. They are no longer bedbound but are moving toward being off the ventilator and toward improved health status. Depression and delirium are common with bedbound patients. They almost lose their sense of self. Mobilization provides these patients with a sense of hope that they are progressing (Peterson, 2011).

THE ELDERLY AND IMMOBILITY

The elderly greatly benefit from mobility and although not all can reach independence, many can improve their quality of life. Moving from one position to another is the first step. Mobility is increased in increments—from changing position in bed, to transferring to a chair, then to a wheelchair, to walking with an assistive device, to independence if possible. These steps increase independence and reduce admission to long-term care. The elderly who participate in mobility protocols are often able to do many self-care activities.

The elderly can quickly become deconditioned in the hospital. Functional decline can occur as early as the second day of hospitalization for elderly adults. If an elderly person is on bed rest, the decline can come quickly. If they become too weak to be discharged to home, they may need to go to a nursing home for further recovery. The fact is that the majority of older patients want to go directly home from the hospital. Simple interventions such as having patients sit out of bed for meals or walking with them several times a day increase their strength and mobility.

One program aimed at preventing health decline in the hospitalized elderly is the NICHE program. This program was developed by the Hartford Institute at the New York University College of Nursing. It is a national program that focuses on the needs of hospitalized older adults. NICHE specifically relies on protocols that assist the patient to prevent complications that can occur in the hospital. These needs normally fall into an established set of symptoms that are seen more often in older patients. Geriatric resource nurses are educated to the changes in the elderly that can lead to serious health problems. These changes include delirium and memory loss, falls, pain control, nutrition, multiple medications, and issues pertaining to skin, incontinence, and sleep (Middlesex Hospital's community e-newsletter, 2011).

Specific activities can prevent decline in the hospitalized elderly. Using incidental activities as part of the daily routine can promote some independence. Some activities include:

- Having patients walk to the bathroom or toilet if possible rather than using the commode
- Encourage patients to participate in care and basic hygiene, washing the parts of the body they can reach
- Have patient sit out of bed as soon as possible
- Eat meals out of bed if able
- Involve physical therapy/occupational therapy in care activities
- Ambulate patients outside of their room if able
- Offer patients toileting on a consistent basis

Increasing patient's mobility in long-term care can expand on those activities initiated while in acute care. Activities aimed at keeping the mind and body sharp can assist in increasing independence as much as possible. Patients should not only sit out of bed for meals but if possible join others for meals. Group activities and exercise not only increase strength but also increase socialization. Physical therapy should include methods to progress in mobility—simple standing and transfers, leading to band training and walking with an assistive device, to as independent as possible.

Though not all patients will achieve independence, increasing mobility has multiple effects. Falls are reduced and patients are safer. They have increased attention span and can socialize with others. In addition their body strength is improved, improving circulation, respirations, and cardiovascular status. Their skin maintains integrity; it is supple and receives appropriate nutrients (Victorian Government Health Information, 2012).

Increasing mobility in the home is also important. Regular activity combined with a thoughtfully designed "safe" living environment can help the elderly live independently for as long as possible. Exercise is just as important for older people as it is for people at any stage of life. All older individuals can benefit from a regular exercise program. Regular exercise and activity keep the body strong. Blood pressure is lowered and glucose use by the body is controlled. Studies by the National Institutes of Health have shown that exercise is the best way to increase mobility in the elderly. Though everyone is at a different level, activities can be developed to increase activity. Using a multidisciplinary team, a plan can be developed to increase the level of activity in the homebound elderly (Victorian Government Health Information, 2012).

FAST FACTS in a NUTSHELL

Assess an elderly person's abilities before starting a mobility program. Include a physician as part of the multidisciplinary team.

MOBILITY PROTOCOLS IN CRITICAL CARE UNITS

The effect of patient immobility has already been discussed. Not only does it affect the physical well-being of patients, it also affects their psychological well-being. The patient is usually most immobile when he or she is in the critical care unit. This basic need is often ignored simply because of the magnitude of care a patient may require. Progressive mobility for patients who are in critical care, even those who are on mechanical ventilation, is safe, prevents complications of immobility, and is cost-effective.

Progressive mobility protocols are evidence based and follow specific practices. It is not simply getting a patient up; it is getting a patient up at the most appropriate time for the patient. Care for the individual patient is planned so that mobility is an integral part of it. This is a team approach that includes but is not limited to physical and occupational therapy, nursing, respiratory therapy, the critical care physician, and midlevel staff. The protocol is best if it becomes part of the standard of care for the unit and follows the patient when he or she progresses to another area (Agency for Healthcare Research and Quality, 2012).

Because the effects of immobility begin the first day in intensive care, the patient's abilities are assessed initially and on a routine basis—usually every 8 to 12 hours. Patients that are at high risk for complications due to immobility are then progressed through specific steps. If the steps are not met, the protocol is not discontinued but rather the patient is assessed at a later time. Patients' tolerance based on their heart rate changes, blood pressure, and oxygenation are assessed at regular increments.

In some ICU patients, simple changes in position are not tolerated by the body. These patients may need to be evaluated frequently. Just as small position shifts can help in offloading pressure, they can also help with other complications of mobility.

Sample Mobility Protocol

1. Range of motion exercises and small shifts in position to full repositioning as tolerated
2. Elevate head of bed 30 to 45 degrees
3. Head of bed elevated 45 degrees and legs in dependent position in recliner chair
4. Head of bed to 65 degrees and legs in full dependent position in chair
5. Head of bed to 65 degrees and feet on floor
6. Stand or pivot to chair, tolerate out of bed for increased increments
7. Ambulate and increase tolerance as able

Each step is done for a specific amount of time, at least 30 minutes before progressing. The patient's tolerance is documented not only subjectively but also specifically by heart rate, blood pressure, and other measures based on condition. In conjunction with mobility, patients on ventilators are also often placed on a weaning program. Early weaning programs also decrease complications for the patient (King, 2012).

FAST FACTS in a NUTSHELL

When increasing a patient's mobility, it is important to protect the patient's skin. Assist the patient to move carefully. If the patient is going to be sitting up in a chair for a period of time, ensure the patient has a pressure-relieving surface to sit on.

Increasing a patient's mobility is important in all settings. It is a basic care need that often is not done due to other care needed by the patient. Decreasing or preventing complications of immobility, however, helps the patient progress to a different level of care. This not only helps the patient but it helps the facility by decreasing the cost of care at the higher level. It also helps the nurses by improving patient outcomes whenever possible.

Pressure ulcer prevention is just one benefit from increasing patient mobility. Mobility increases circulation and therefore increases blood flow to the skin. Patients in all settings do well when they are able to reach their maximum potential. The next sections will discuss continued aspects of pressure ulcer prevention followed by what to do if an ulcer does occur.

8

Go to the Mattress: Mattresses and Specialty Beds

Surfaces that can prevent, help reduce, or relieve pressure are often discussed in health care settings and are often very confusing. Pressure redistribution surfaces or support surfaces are used to offload pressure on soft tissue. Appropriate surfaces manage pressure load to tissues, moisture, microclimate, friction, and shear. The goal is obtaining the best pressure distribution possible rather than just on one part of the body (Lyder, 2008). There is a body of literature that supports the use of pressure redistribution in preventing pressure ulcers. Essentially anything can reduce pressure. So it is important to clearly identify what type of mattress is being used for patient care.

Upon completion of this chapter, the reader will be able to:

1. Define pressure reduction and pressure relief as they refer to specialty mattresses and support surfaces
2. Identify the types of specialty beds/mattresses and key functions of each
3. Discuss reimbursement strategies for specialty beds/mattresses

PRESSURE REDUCTION VERSUS PRESSURE RELIEF

There are essentially two types of surfaces—pressure relieving and pressure reducing. *Pressure-relieving mattresses* are those that are the best for prevention as pressure is relieved. *Pressure-reducing mattresses*, on the other hand, reduce pressure and are minimally effective in preventing and treating pressure ulcers. What is important is that pressure to bony prominences is reduced below the capillary closing pressure (32 mmHg). This measure is a standard gauge when evaluating or choosing a support surface for a patient or as a standard in a facility. Essentially the pressure from the surface does not place additional stress on the body's tissues (Sslcido & Lorenzo, 2012).

There are many types of mattresses from various manufacturers, but none have been identified as superior to others. Some have better features or have been used successfully but no single manufacturer has been identified as better than another. What is important is that the use of a support surface is effective in preventing pressure ulcers as compared to a regular mattress. Support surfaces can be powered or nonpowered (National Pressure Advisory Panel, 2009). The Centers for Medicare and Medicaid (CMS) separates the types of pressure distribution:

Group I: Static surfaces that do not require electricity. They include air, foam, gel, or water in the form of overlays or mattresses. These mattresses are used for patients at lower risk for pressure ulcer development.

Group II: Mattresses powered by electricity and are dynamic in nature. These mattresses are alternating and low air loss mattresses. These devices are used with patients who have pressure ulcers or who are at a moderate to high risk for developing them.

Group III: Air fluidized beds. Silicone-coated beads are contained in the mattress; these beads liquefy in response to the air pumped through them. These beds are used for high-risk patients with multiple pressure ulcers (Lyder, 2008; Wound Ostomy and

Continence Nurses Society [WOCN], 2010). These beds at times are cumbersome and the expense may be prohibitive.

The question then is what is the best surface or mattress to use? It is clear that the choice depends on the patient status and need. However, it may also come down to economics. What will the patient's insurance pay for? In this case, the simplest mattress may be the choice. The most important thing to remember is that, as with any mattress, repositioning is necessary. In the home, family members may need to be taught to move patients frequently and effectively no matter what the surface. This is also important in acute or long-term care. Positioning is necessary without shortcuts (WOCN, 2010).

PAYMENT FOR SUPPORT SURFACES

So what does insurance cover? Of course insurance companies vary but all require specific documentation of the needs of the individual. Documentation that is in the patient's chart follows the standard of care from any conservative measures taken to the need for more complex treatment. A patient usually qualifies for insurance coverage (based on Medicare guidelines) if he or she meets the following:

Group I: The patient is completely immobile (cannot make changes in body position by himself or herself) or the patient has limited mobility with either impaired nutritional status, fecal or urinary incontinence, altered sensory perception, or compromised circulatory status.

Group II: The patient has multiple Stage II pressure ulcers on the trunk or pelvis, has been part of a comprehensive pressure ulcer prevention program for at least 30 days, and the ulcers have worsened or have not changed in that time period; or the patient has large or multiple Stage III or IV pressure ulcers on the trunk or pelvis; or the patient has had a myocutaneous skin graft or flap on the trunk or pelvis within the past 2 months; or the patient was on a support surface prior to recent discharge from a hospital or nursing facility (United Seating and Mobility, 2012).

When referring to these guidelines, it is clear that the patient is in need and what the needs are. Careful documentation can truly benefit the patient. All caregivers need to be on the same page. If patients are debilitated and are at risk for pressure ulcer development, they should be part of a pressure ulcer prevention program in every setting. The above prevention methods are easy to accomplish whether in the most advanced acute care setting or in the home.

=======*FAST FACTS in a NUTSHELL*

Assessing and reassessing the patient on a regular basis to determine whether the surface he or she is on is adequate or should be discontinued benefits all involved. This not only provides the best surface for the patient but is also cost-effective.

CHOICE OF SUPPORT SURFACE

When choosing a support surface it is important to tailor the product to the patient. Specific guidelines for use can ensure that the patient receives the best surface for his or her skin status. This is also cost-effective for the facility or individual patient (Sslcido & Lorenzo, 2012).

In acute care there are three general rules when choosing a support surface for a patient:

1. Static (pressure-relieving or -reducing) mattresses are usually sufficient if the patient's skin is frail and/or the patient has a minor Stage II or Stage I pressure ulcer or less. These patients should be able to be repositioned easily or can assist in repositioning.

2. Dynamic (low air loss or air fluidized [pressure relieving]) mattresses are utilized for patients who have a complicated Stage II ulcer or greater. These patients need to be repositioned and cannot do so themselves.
3. Multipositioning or active support surfaces are used for patients who have complicated Stage IV ulcers or who have had skin grafting. These patients cannot turn themselves and cannot have pressure on the affected area.

TABLE 8.1 Analysis of Basic Support Surfaces

Surface	Advantage	Disadvantage
Air mattress/ overlay	Low maintenance Inexpensive Patient can use in home or in facility Low tech and easy to use Single patient use; patients can take with them	Need method to inflate Can be punctured Proper inflation must be ensured to prevent bottoming out Can add additional height to the mattress and become a fall risk
Gel mattress/ overlay	Low maintenance Resists puncture Easy to clean and can be used on multiple surfaces including operating room table or emergency department stretcher Durable	Can be heavy to transport It is important to ensure gel is effective; need to check manufacturer for life of product Can be expensive Little documented research regarding its effectiveness
Foam mattress/ overlay	Lightweight No puncturing Can tear No maintenance Single-patient use and can be used in any environment	Holds moisture and heat Fragile, use is limited Cannot clean May retain odors/ bacteria
Water mattress/ bed/overlay	Common material Easy to clean Can be cooling; however, it does require heating unit	Requires heating unit Heavy Cannot transfer patient easily High maintenance

(continued)

TABLE 8.1 Analysis of Basic Support Surfaces (*continued*)

Surface	Advantage	Disadvantage
Dynamic overlays	Easy to clean Controls moisture and microclimate Deflates to ease transfers Pump is reusable Patient can use in any setting	Can be punctured Produce noise Power source necessary Higher tech as they need some assembly Can add height to current mattress causing fall risk
Replacement pressure-relieving mattress	Used for all patients No decision tree Staff time reduced Easy to clean Low maintenance Mattresses now reduce friction and shear as well as control moisture	High cost initially It is important to replace per manufacturers' recommendation as they may lose effectiveness Higher cost mattress may be necessary to include moisture control and friction and shear
Low air loss bed	Controls allow for assist in positioning; head and feet can be elevated Reduces friction and shear Controls moisture May have cooling effect	Requires electricity source May be difficult to use in home Expensive and requires setup Often rented, creating extra steps for staff It may be difficult to assist patient out of bed, even deflated Patient must be assisted to position Noisy
Air fluidized bed	Lowest interface pressure, relieves pressure consistently Reduces friction and shear Reduces moisture	Heavy Because of the moisture, balance can actually cause dehydration or fluid and electrolyte imbalance Creates warm climate Difficult to transfer and help patient out of bed, decreasing mobility

Source: Agency for Healthcare Research and Quality, 2010; Dorner, 2009; Salcido & Lorenzo, 2012.

Using the descriptions in Table 8.1, the nurse can choose the appropriate surface for the patient. In addition, documentation of patient findings will only support the needs of the patient. It is in this manner that insurance companies will approve the appropriate surface and therefore the patient will get the appropriate care. (See Appendix II for major types of surfaces on the market and manufacturers.)

REPLACEMENT MATTRESSES

There has been a recent trend toward replacing all mattresses in a facility with pressure-relieving mattresses. This is an expensive undertaking but is worth the cost in the long run. These mattresses provide pressure relief and friction and shear prevention, as well as moisture control. In acute care this may be especially important due to the many different patients with many different issues. As already discussed, young people can develop pressure ulcers simply by not moving or being unable to move easily due to pain. Replacing all mattresses also eliminates the need to decide what type of mattress to use for the patient. A patient will then have a low air loss or fluidized bed if he or she has a complicated Stage II or above. Other patients will do well with the standard pressure-relieving mattress.

Replacement mattresses often are a mix of gel and foam, making them light and easy to use. They are easy to clean and have multipatient use. Manufacturers will determine the life of the mattress. It is important to maintain this life expectancy to ensure the mattress is effective. If the mattress is not replaced at the appropriate time, pressure ulcers can occur if the mattresses bottom out or lose their pressure-relieving abilities. There are many mattresses on the market. *The best mattress has a warranty, is cost-effective, and has prevention of friction and shear as well as moisture control. The mattresses should also be comfortable as well as not increasing the risk to the patient due to added height or slippery fabric.* (See Appendix II for replacement mattresses on the market and manufacturers.)

MATTRESSES/SUPPORT SURFACES IN THE HOME

In the home-care setting the nurse may need to consider the condition of the mattresses patients are using. Even with positioning, old or worn-out mattresses could actually cause ulcers. Some old mattresses have creases, may be made of plastic, or may simply not be supportive. Pressure ulcers are truly prevented by pressure redistribution. In place of the old mattress, considering mattresses that relieve pressure would be the best scenario. Patients in home care may also be using older mattresses. If the patient is bedbound or spends a good portion of time in bed, a hospital bed or overlay would be of benefit. Again, appropriate assessment and documentation of patient needs could greatly affect the patient. A simple survey of what the patient is using could have a positive outcome.

In order for payment from the CMS (most insurance companies follow these guidelines) for support surface or specialty mattress reimbursement, specific requirements must be met:

- Detailed and written order from a physician
- Information from the physician regarding diagnosis
- Any written documentation concerning the need for the surface
- Specific and detailed medical record documentation
- Proof of delivery and receipt of the product

In addition a care plan for the patient must be established that includes routine care, assessment, and reassessment of need. The surface will continue to be used until the ulcer is healed. It is very difficult to continue with the same surface especially if it is high in cost. If the ulcer is healed, in general the patient will be downgraded to a lower-level surface or no surface at all depending on need and appropriate documentation (CMS, 2012).

CHAIR SURFACES

Remember the 2-hour guideline: A pressure ulcer can develop in that brief a time frame especially if the patient is sitting in a chair without padding or pressure relief. Chairs that are upholstered or look soft can fool the caregiver into believing that it is a support surface and acceptable for the patient to be in for long periods. However, pressure redistribution is just as important when a patient is seated in a chair as when in a bed.

When a person is in a chair for a period of time, the constant pressure against the skin reduces blood flow to areas of contact. Skin begins to break down and the tissue dies. Friction and shear—caused by sliding down in the chair, or being moved improperly from a stretcher to a bed—can make the problem worse (Institute for Healthcare Improvement, 2011). Patients in wheelchairs often have friction and shear injuries on the backs of the thighs. These injuries are classic when someone is sitting in a chair and is not stable in that chair.

Just as with support surfaces for the bed, there are many companies that make support surfaces for chairs. No one type stands out as better than the others but use of a support surface for the chair is important for patients who are at high risk or for those who have pressure ulcers. Studies have found that patients prone to pressure ulcers and who sit in wheelchairs are at high risk for ulcer development if they do not have a support surface (Brienza, 2010). In addition, patients that are constantly sliding out of a wheelchair can have serious damage to their skin. Increasing mobility has already been discussed as important but it is also important to consider the patient's skin when the patient is sitting out of bed. The facility or patient may find it prudent to custom fit a chair to a patient rather than pay the cost of a pressure ulcer (Institute for Healthcare Improvement, 2011).

In the acute care setting, simple air-filled chair overlays have been found to be beneficial to patients that are at risk or who already have pressure ulcers. These overlays alternate pressure through the movement of air in the cushion. These pads are relatively inexpensive and can be used for all patients. They also come in a size for bariatric patients. Patients who are in a critical care or rehabilitative setting may benefit from a higher-end chair cushion such as those made in the same manner as pressure-relief mattresses.

═══════════════════════════════════*FAST FACTS in a NUTSHELL*

Caregivers should be taught to use inexpensive chair cushions for all patients who are out of bed for any length of time. If the patient is debilitated or has serious skin breakdown, a different cushion may be necessary but simple prevention methods go a long way.

(See Appendix III: Chair Services Available and Manufacturers)

PART

III

Pressure Ulcer Treatment

9

What Happens When a Patient Does Acquire a Pressure Ulcer?

Pressure ulcers do occur at times as the skin is an organ and organs do fail or die. Given the human condition and patients who do not choose to follow health advice, pressure ulcers may develop. As a health care professional it must be remembered and documented that everything possible has been done to prevent the ulcer from occurring. Pressure ulcers are reasonably avoidable. Simple prevention strategies have been proven to prevent ulcers from occurring. Nurses can provide what is best for their patients and maintain appropriate skin integrity. However, if a patient has a pressure ulcer or one develops, it is important to choose the appropriate treatment modalities to ensure the ulcer improves or does not worsen.

Upon completion of this chapter, the reader will be able to:

1. Determine if an ulcer is caused by pressure
2. Successfully document findings related to an ulcer
3. Appropriately assess a wound and surrounding skin

IDENTIFYING THE CAUSE OF A PRESSURE ULCER: IS IT TRULY PRESSURE?

The Centers for Medicare and Medicaid Services (CMS) has specific guidelines in relation to patients acquiring pressure ulcers after they enter a facility. According to the regulations a patient should not attain a pressure ulcer in a facility. That facility must do everything possible to prevent the ulcer from occurring. The only exception is if the patient's clinical condition changes. These ulcers can be said to be *unavoidable* (Black, 2011). Patients acquire unavoidable pressure ulcers if they are hemodynamically unstable and require vasopressive medications or mechanical support to maintain blood pressure or cardiac output. In these patients, turning may not be possible and shifts in weight are not sufficient to prevent blood vessels from constricting. Patients who are critically unstable may have organ failure, including the skin (Black, 2011). Documenting patient status carefully is important to essentially prove the case of an unavoidable pressure ulcer.

Patients who are dying may acquire *Kennedy terminal ulcers*. These ulcers are characterized by purple pear-shaped ulcers usually on the buttocks, sacrum, or gluteal cleft. They usually occur approximately 2 days before death (Black, 2011). Kennedy terminal ulcers occur quickly and when they do occur it is evident. Often these patients are on comfort measures and it is not essential that they are moved frequently. The goal and plan of care focus on comfort, pain control, and protection.

A patient's skin can be damaged in many ways. Friction and shear can remove the top layer of skin; these two forces in combination can cause a pressure ulcer. Frail skin can tear easily and the damage associated with moisture can be painful and devastating. Wounds on the lower extremities can be from poor vascular or arterial status. Even at pressure sites, different types of wounds can occur. Therefore it behooves the nurse to know what caused the patient's ulcer. Is it pressure?

Clear identification of wound type is needed not only for reimbursement purposes but also for the safety of the patient and in order to choose the appropriate care. Education about pressure ulcer staging is important for all caregivers. Everyone should have an understanding of and be able to identify ulcers that are caused by pressure. Of course sometimes even the trained eye is unsure of the cause of an ulcer. Then careful discussion and observation of the wound are needed. If there is any doubt how the wound occurred and it has the location and characteristics of a pressure ulcer, then it needs to be documented as such and reported to CMS.

When caring for a patient who has many lines and tubes in the body, the effect of these tubes on the skin needs to be monitored. Tubes that are left on the skin or pressed between body parts can cause a pressure ulcer. If the skin is thin at a pressure site, the ulcer can cause serious problems as it may be down to the bone quickly. Ensure lines and medical devices are away from the body (European Pressure Ulcer Advisory Panel [EPUAP] & the National Pressure Ulcer Advisory Panel [NPUAP], 2009).

═══════════════════════════*FAST FACTS in a NUTSHELL*

Patients that have frail skin can acquire a pressure ulcer on any part of the body. Assess all tubes and lines carefully. Even the most basic medical equipment can cause serious skin issues.

WOUND ASSESSMENT AND DOCUMENTATION

Just as careful documentation is needed on admission and for risk assessment, so is documentation about an existing wound. Assessing a wound includes careful descriptions about all aspects of the wound. The wound is assessed on discovery and weekly thereafter. Regular assessment of the wound will provide information about the wound status; that is, if it is healing, if it is infected, or if the current treatment is appropriate (DeMarco, n.d.).

Specific standardized methods of documentation are important to wound assessment. The following are general guidelines for accurate documentation.

Location

Carefully describe the location of the wound. The correct anatomical terms are the most appropriate as everyone will know exactly where the wound is. What pressure point?

Description/Staging

Follow the NPUAP guidelines for staging. Wounds are not back staged; they are staged as they are found. If the wound is identified as a Stage III, it will always be a Stage III but a healing or granulating Stage III (Wound Ostomy and Continence Nurses Society [WOCN], 2011).

═══════════════════════════*FAST FACTS in a NUTSHELL*

Staff members and caregivers should be taught to describe the wound as clearly as possible. Even if they have difficulty determining the stage/classification, this documentation will be evident in the patient's medical record and can help in determining the plan of care for the patient.

Measurement

There are various modalities for wound measurement. The most common, and often the most accurate, is by using a head-to-toe landmark for length and a hip-to-hip landmark for width. Like assessment, wounds are measured once per week (e.g., measure every Monday). Everyone assessing a wound will do so in the same manner for accuracy and so that the next person knows exactly what is occurring with the wound. Measuring tapes should be readily available and all caregivers should be educated about their correct use. Wounds are always measured in centimeters (cm).

Length: Measure the longest portion of the wound using the top of the head and the feet as landmarks.

Width: The widest portion is measured using each hip as a landmark.

Depth: A premoistened cotton-tipped applicator is inserted gently into the deepest part of the wound. Measure from the tip of the applicator to the skin level and use the measuring ruler for determination.

Undermining: Using another cotton-tipped applicator, assess if the wound undermines (is larger surrounding the primary wound site, often occurs at the edges). Identify undermining using a clock for location; for example, *"The wound does have undermining, which measures 1 cm from 3 o'clock to 12 o'clock."*

═══════════════════════════════════════ *FAST FACTS in a NUTSHELL*

When wounds are packed with dressings, it is important to do so gently and minimally. Forcing a large amount of dressing into a wound can actually damage the wound, sometimes causing undermining.

Tunneling: Use another cotton-tipped applicator to measure if the wound has a deeper or tunneling portion. Measure to the skin and use a ruler to determine depth.

== *FAST FACTS in a NUTSHELL*

If there is a tunnel or deeper section of the wound, it is necessary to apply or pack dressings into this area as well. If this area does not heal, it will always be open and can become infected or reopen the wound.

Wound Base Appearance

The description of the wound base tells about the wound status. What does it look like—color, tissue appearance? Is it clean or is there debris within it?

Review of Wound Healing

- Under normal healing a wound that is acute will go through three phases: inflammatory (4 to 6 days), proliferative (3 days to 3 weeks), and remodeling (2 weeks to 2 years).
- Basically when the wound is new, it is flooded with inflammatory cells that clean the wound.
- During the proliferative stage there is protein and extracellular matrix building.
- In the remodeling phase, collagen is produced to strengthen the wound.
- Chronic wounds do not go through the same building and remodeling.
- Large wounds if not closed in surgery heal from the bottom up.
- Acute wounds such as surgical wounds are closed and must heal by *secondary intention*.
- Sometimes wounds are left open initially and there is a delay in closure. These wounds heal by *tertiary intention*.

(EPUAP and NPUAP, 2009).

The tissue within a wound varies. The healthiest wound will have pink granulation tissue, which indicates the wound is getting stronger and is building. If there is other tissue within the wound, it will have to be removed (debrided) in order for cells to continue to move within the wound. Scars are not as strong and the area will never have the same strength as regular tissue. This is why a patient who has healed pressure ulcers is always protected because these areas can easily open. When documenting tissue in the wound, it is usually documented in percentages; for example, *"There was 10% yellow slough in the wound."*

Tissue within a wound includes:

Granulation—Tissue appears pink or red and usually looks grainy and moist. It is the connective tissue that forms in major wounds during healing. It consists of new blood cells, epithelium, myoblasts, and a cell matrix.

Necrotic tissue—Appears gray or black, and can be moist or dry. It is essentially dead tissue within the wound or covering the wound.

Eschar—Appears as a thick scar or hard crust covering a wound. In a sensitive area such as the heel, eschar is usually left in place as it is the body's protective covering. However, if the patient is able to ambulate and this tissue is impeding ambulation, it may have to be removed. In order for a wound to heal, eschar needs to be removed.

Slough—Appears yellow or white and may be stringy in appearance. This too can impede wound healing and will need to be removed

Epithelialization—Appears as new or shiny tissue that grows in from edges of the wound surface. The wound is beginning to resurface.

(EPUAP and NPUAP, 2009)

Drainage/Exudate

In assessing wound drainage, look at the old dressing. Depending on when it was changed last, it will determine how much drainage or exudate is in a wound. The desired drainage is bloody to serous, usually a moderate or small amount depending on the size of the wound. Exudate is another gauge of wound healing. Purulent drainage with an odor most likely means infection. Wounds that are acute will have more drainage; chronic wounds generally not.

All chronic wounds are contaminated with bacteria. The bacteria, however, do not take over the tissue (colonization). This is why taking a wound culture is not really needed unless there are signs of infection. Signs of infection include redness, inflammation, pus, and odor. All wounds do have an odor but it should not permeate the room. If a culture is warranted, the wound should be cleansed first. The drainage itself is not swabbed; rather, swab different parts of the wound.

Wounds that are stalled may look pink but may actually be colonized and have a bioburden resistant to antibiotics. These wounds appear pink but flat, not grainy or moist. Debridement or removal of foreign matter in such wounds may be necessary, which will be discussed later.

Wound Edges

Wound edges can be defined or not defined; that is, the wound can be irregular in shape. The edges should be evident and attached to the sides of the wound. If the edges are rolled (epibole) the wound is not healing properly and may need surgical intervention. Edges that are white or macerated are too moist. Edges that are calloused or fibrotic are also not healing well and may need to be debrided.

Appearance of the Surrounding Skin or Peri-Wound

The skin surrounding the wound should be healthy. A pink color (erythema) may be normal especially if the wound is in the early phases. At a later time there should be minimal color surrounding the wound. If there is edema and purulent drainage, infection should be considered. Just as with wound edges, peri-wound skin that is macerated indicates the skin is too moist. A change in treatment may be necessary or the skin may need to be protected.

Pain

People experience pain in different ways. Some have high tolerance for pain while others experience pain at the slightest movement. Wounds that are shallow are typically more painful than those that are deeper because of the location of nerves. Consider that nerve endings are in the dermis, which underlies the top layer or epidermis. Ensuring that patients are comfortable when doing a dressing change is essential. Medication is offered prior to dressing change and observation about how the patient tolerates the change is also done. New onset of pain may mean the wound is infected and the wound should be assessed carefully (Dziedzic, 2011).

Careful wound assessment is essential to determine treatment. The description provides a picture of the wound. This picture allows all care providers to know what is happening with the wound. In addition the assessment is done regularly and also documented. This documentation also provides validation of the care the patient needs that, as already discussed, is necessary for insurance payment. The next step for wound care is to choose the appropriate treatment, which will be discussed in the next sections.

10

Treatment:
Creating an Environment of Healing

The treatment of pressure ulcers actually depends on the type of ulcer. For pressure ulcers, if the wound is shallow the goal is to promote growth and protect the ulcer from damage. Often no dressing is needed except for the use of a barrier cream. Deeper wounds such as Stage II ulcers require tissue growth to heal, while very deep wounds such as Stage III or IV ulcers need granulation and epithelialization (contraction). The goal of treatment is also a factor: If the goal is palliative, then comfort and protection may be the only treatment provided. The treatment therefore depends on the ulcer and the patient's health status.

Upon completion of this chapter, the reader will be able to:

1. Choose a particular dressing or treatment
2. Identify two types of dressings and the use for each
3. Identify two types of adjunct therapies used for wound healing

THE BASICS OF CHOOSING
THE APPROPRIATE DRESSING

There are several considerations when choosing a wound dressing. A primary factor is who will be doing the dressing change. Can the patient do it himself or herself, or will someone else need to be taught? Is the dressing appropriate for a caregiver to change? Another concern is resources: Is the patient able to afford the dressing or will it be covered by insurance? The care for the patient is multidisciplinary so social workers or case managers may have to be consulted. Health care insurance companies are often very good at determining cost and what will be covered. Many have registered nurses with whom care can be discussed. Some insurance companies use particular manufacturers or brands for dressings and treatments and there may be confusion on discharge. Determination of what is going to be used for the patient should be made before discharge, if possible.

Wounds epithelialize when there is a moist environment. Cells require moisture to grow across the wound bed from the wound edges. If the wound is dry, cells must find a moist area in order to progress. There are many recent developments in wound dressings and there are many choices. The primary goals of wound dressings are to promote rapid healing, protect the wound, and decrease pain. Dressings are changed as infrequently as possible to meet these goals.

Wounds are assessed with each dressing change and, as already indicated, measured at least once a week. As the wound changes so does the dressing. If a wound is draining heavily, a dressing to contain that drainage would be appropriate. However, once the drainage decreases, moisture may need to be added. That is when nurses use keen assessment skills to achieve the best patient outcomes.

Dressings may be dictated by the institution but may not be the most cost-effective choice. Acute care facilities like home care and long-term care have limited dollars. Therefore, no matter what the setting, the least expensive, simplest dressing may be the best choice. This may also be the best for the patient in the long run. Wound outcomes need to be patient centric and realistic (Baranoski, 2012).

There are four basic guidelines when choosing the appropriate dressing for a wound:

1. If the wound is draining heavily, drainage must be contained and surrounding skin protected.
2. If the wound is dry, moisture must be added as moisture is necessary for cell growth.
3. If there is dead space within a wound, it must be filled with dressing.
4. If there is dead tissue in the wound, it must be removed or the wound will not heal (DeMarco, n.d.).

TYPES OF DRESSINGS

(See Appendix IV for dressings on the market and the manufacturers.)

Antimicrobials (Topical)

There are several forms of topical antimicrobial ointments, creams, instillations, or dressings. Topical antimicrobials should be used in cases of infection—wound pain, foul odor, purulent drainage, or fever. They can also be used in high-risk patients or wounds (such as burns) to prevent infections. There are many theories that suggest antimicrobials have aided in the development of resistant bacteria. But the most important thing is that they be used according to the manufacturer's recommendation. In general, they are to be used for no longer than a 2-week period. If used longer, the medication can begin to harm the good tissue.

There has been some controversy regarding silver-impregnated dressings. The goal of the dressings is to reduce the bioburden (microorganism growth). Healing comes from cell growth; antimicrobials are used to prevent infection. They promote wound healing by providing a clean noninfected wound but may not be necessary (Katz, 2012).

Similarly, the use of Dakin's solution in wound care has been controversial. Dakin's solution is a mixture of sodium hypochlorite and boric acid—it certainly has a chlorine-like smell. Through experience it has cleansed some foul-smelling wounds with thick drainage. The guide for this is to use the weakest solution possible (commonly 0.125% to 0.25% is ordered). It is effective against multiple anaerobic and aerobic organisms. It is also effective against fungus (Arnold-Lolng, 2010). The guideline for antimicrobials is to use Dakin's for as short a course as possible, again generally no longer than 2 weeks.

Alginates

Alginates are derived from seaweed and are highly absorbable. They are also biodegradable and can be left in the wound. These dressings conform to the wound and are absorbent. The gel that is formed as these products absorb exudate forms a moist covering over the slough, preventing it from drying out. These dressings require moisture to function correctly, so alginates are not indicated for dry wounds or those covered with hard necrotic tissue. There are sheets made of alginate fiber for shallow wounds with heavy exudate, while rope or ribbon alginate can be packed inside of the cavity of a wound.

Barriers

Barrier creams, powders, or films protect the surrounding skin of a wound or frail skin to prevent further damage.

Barriers can be used for shallow superficial wounds creating a protective cover. They are also used for patients with moisture-associated skin damage to protect the skin from urine or feces even if there are superficial open areas.

Collagen

Collagen stimulates wound repair and epithelial cell activity. The use of collagen in wounds is multifaceted as it controls moisture. The dressing is usually inserted within the wound. There are a number of different collagen dressings available that are combined with agents such as gels, pastes, polymers, and oxidized regenerated cellulose. Most collagen dressings contain collagen derived from bovine and porcine sources. Although these collagens are purified, there remains a concern regarding the potential for contamination or the spread of disease from the animal source. Human-derived collagens are linked with fewer concerns but they are expensive, which may prohibit their use. There has been recent work with fish collagen for dressings.

Composite Products

Composite dressings are made up of layers that usually consist of a nonadhering layer, an absorbent layer, and a moisture-vapor permeable layer. They often have a nonadhering border that allows the dressing to stay in place. Usually, they are composed of multiple layers and incorporate a semi- or nonadherent pad that covers the wound. They can function as either a primary or a secondary dressing on a wide variety of wounds and may be used with topical medications. New dressings with a silicone component can be used for protection but must also be lifted carefully to assess the wound underneath or to apply topical treatment. They are usually changed every 3 to 5 days depending on the policy of the facility.

Foams

Foam dressings are usually made from polyurethane and are highly absorbent. The foam dressings prevent the maceration of surrounding skin. It is often used as a cover dressing. They are very good for wounds with heavy exudate. There are also modalities that can be used for deep cavity wounds as packing to collect drainage and maintain a moist environment. They are also good for weeping ulcers.

Gauze

Gauze is simple to use and is available in multiple forms—pads, dressings, and rolls. Gauze is commonly used as a protectant for surgical wounds. The use of wet to dry saline gauze dressings has been used for many years and they have been debated for just as long. The goal of a wet to dry saline dressing is to debride especially if placed in the wound very wet. When the dressing is removed from the wound, the bad tissue comes out with it. Unfortunately the good skin also comes with it. Generally, dressings are now placed in the wound moist; this keeps the wound itself moist and allows for the drainage to be absorbed.

Hydrocolloids

Hydrocolloid dressings are made of cellulose and pectin. These are absorbent but yet maintain the wound environment. They are often used as a protectant at a bony prominence. The manufacturer of these dressings usually provides guidelines but in general the dressings are cut larger than the wound. When removing, pull the dressing away from the skin in a taffy-pulling fashion. If the dressing is not cut larger than the wound, they have a tendency to roll.

Nurses often are critical of hydrocolloid dressings as they are difficult to remove and the drainage often forms a thick odorous ball, which is actually cleaning the wound. If removed gently they should cause no damage to surrounding tissue. Usually the dressings are left in place for 3 to 5 days depending on the policy of the facility. There is also often a strong odor when removed but this is the old tissue underneath.

Hydrofiber

Hydrofiber dressings are highly absorbent, even more so than alginates, but they need to be removed from the wound. There are now dressings with fiber in them so that they can be removed easily. Like alginates, they are absorptive and require a cover dressing. They are made up of carboxymethylcellulose and are conformable. These dressings absorb a large amount of exudate and transform into a soft gel creating a moist, healing environment. They are rinsed from the wound with saline and remove some dead tissue in the process without damaging new tissue.

Hydrogels

Hydrogels replace moisture in the wound and often are said to feel soothing. They are usually used in shallow wounds to promote growth and to protect. Hydrogels come as a gel or in sheets. They are formulations of water, polymers, and other ingredients with no shape, designed to donate moisture to a dry wound and to maintain a moist healing environment. They have a high moisture content that serves to rehydrate wound tissue. Hydrogels also provide some debridement and can be used on full or partial thickness wounds and wounds with necrosis. They can be as soothing as a gel and can be used for radiation burns. Hydrogels usually require a secondary dressing to cover and protect (DeMarco, n.d.).

FAST FACTS in a NUTSHELL

Assess wounds on a regular basis—at least weekly. Ensure everyone describes the wound using standard methods already discussed. Also adjust the dressing type as changes in the wound are noted; for example, changes in exudate or if the wound is moist or dry.

CLEANSING A WOUND PRIOR TO DRESSING APPLICATION

Prior to applying any dressing, cleanse the wound to create the ultimate healing environment. Cleansing the wound assists in removing debris from the wound while protecting delicate tissues. There are many topical wound-cleansing products on the market; however, some such as antiseptics are toxic to tissues especially when used over an extended period of time. Normal saline is safe and inexpensive. It can actually be made in the home.

At-Home Normal Saline Mixture:

- Wash hands and use only clean utensils
- Boil a clean jar and lid for 15 minutes and cool
- Prepare 1 cup water and ½ teaspoon of salt in another clean pot, boiling for 15 minutes
- When cool, place in boiled jar and put on lid without touching the inside of the jar
- Keep only for 24 hours; discard product after this time; use only fresh saline in wound

Cleansing wounds does not mean irrigation. Wounds are gently cleansed by "rinsing" with normal saline. Protect the wound edges and peri-wound skin by drying these areas once cleansing is complete. Cleansing should be done prior to each dressing change. Dressing changes are normally not a sterile procedure for chronic wounds but is done as aseptically as possible. Sterile dressing changes are for serious surgical wounds (such as open chest wounds) or for patients who are immunosuppressed.

Wound irrigation is different from wound cleansing. When irrigating a wound to remove dead tissue, the pressure needs to be high enough to remove the debris. Pressure from 4 to 15 pounds of pressure per square inch (psi) is effective to clean. A 60 mL catheter tip delivers approximately 4.2 psi, while a 35 mL syringe with a large-gauge needle provides 8 psi. The highest irrigation is from a water-pik system, which can be over 50 psi. Irrigation is usually done once a day but may be required more often. Wounds are irrigated based on the wound, patient status, and physician order (Foster, 2013).

Whatever dressing is chosen, the guidelines for dressing choice are used. Whatever treatment is used, it is based on the patient goals. What is expected from the treatment and can the treatment meet the desired result?

ADJUNCT THERAPIES

Wounds and dressing choices are assessed frequently. There are other therapies that may be utilized especially with chronic or nonhealing wounds. Some wounds get stuck in the reaction (inflammatory) phase and may require alternative interventions (Katz, 2012). This is evident when wounds do not change or contract. The wound bed may appear shiny and not have the cobblestone appearance of granulation tissue (Figure 10.1). Adjunct therapies may be necessary.

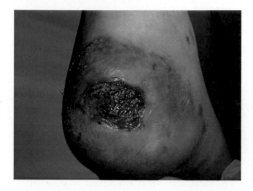

FIGURE 10.1   Stage III pressure ulcer with granulation tissue evident.
Source: National Pressure Ulcer Advisory Panel Resources.

Negative Pressure Wound Therapy (NPWT)

Also called Wound Vac therapy, NPWT creates an environment within the wound to promote wound healing. The NPWT device is essentially a vacuum. A special sponge is inserted into the wound, covered with a transparent drape, and secured to the pump or vacuum. Dressings are foam or gauze and foam with saline added or not. The pressure helps to draw the wound together. It also removes excess fluids and helps promote granulation tissue development (Katz, 2012). Wounds are also protected from the outside environment as the drape is very tight around the wound. Wounds that are appropriate are clean wounds with no more than 25% slough or necrotic tissue in the wound. There also should be no signs of infection in the wound.

Wound Vacs do work very well in helping wounds heal. The cells are able to move freely as warmth and moisture are maintained. The number of sponges inserted in a wound needs to be clearly documented. In addition the usual pressure of the vacuum is set at 125 mm; however, this may not be tolerated by the patient or it may be too high for delicate tissues. The pressure therefore is also documented. If the wound has a high amount of drainage or a lot of sponge inserted, the pressure may be actually placed at 150 mm. The pressure is ordered by the physician.

FAST FACTS in a NUTSHELL

Everyone who touches a Wound Vac should document the same way. Essentially what type of sponge was used, number of sponges, settings, and what the wound looked like. A good method for documentation is to write the number of sponges on the transparent dressing. With this method the number of sponges in the wound is very clear. Sponges have been left in wounds and the wound can quickly heal over them, which can cause serious infection.

Skin Substitutes and Growth Factors

There are other options for wounds that are stalled or recalcitrant. Growth factors such as artificial or laboratory-grown skin and skin substitutes are now commonly available to promote epithelialization and heal chronic wounds (Katz, 2012). These are basically skin grafts that, even when not permanent, can help some wounds to heal. There are a variety of products, each having specific instructions that need to be followed clearly.

Electrical Stimulation (E-STIM) Therapy

E-STIM therapy uses an electrical current that transfers energy into a wound. Like NPWT or skin substitutes, its use can jump-start a wound. It regenerates the wound, reinitiating the processes in inflammation. Electrodes are placed within moist wound beds and the stimulus is away from the body and wound. Care is taken with external skin and the amount of energy needed. Careful documentation is necessary (Katz, 2012).

Hyperbaric Oxygen Therapy

In hyperbaric oxygen therapy the patient is placed in pure oxygen in a pressurized room, a process that has been used for years to relieve decompression issues with scuba divers. This therapy works by increasing the available oxygen to the body's tissue. The blood can carry more oxygen to promote healing. Not everyone is a candidate for hyperbaric oxygen therapy as it does require the patient to be inside of a pressurized chamber. Patients can experience claustrophobia. It can also cause issues with the eardrum or other organs due to the increased pressure and oxygen. Patients are screened very carefully (Mayo Clinic, 2012).

Ultrasound (US)

US is used to increase the elasticity of collagen. It can also decrease muscle stiffness and spasm as well as decreasing pain. US increases oxygen transport to speed up wound healing (Katz, 2012).

Adjunct therapies may be necessary if a patient's wound is not healing. Cost and insurance coverage are often issues. It is usually required to report why traditional therapies did not work or why some other therapy is necessary. Adjunct therapy should be used based on the goals of treating the wound just as with other wound therapies.

11

Debridement of Wounds

Debridement, which is removing dead tissue from the wound, is part of wound management. Removing dead tissue or other material from the wound promotes healing by allowing cells to migrate and granulation to occur (Payne, 2008). Chronic wounds often contain nonviable tissue such as slough. This nonviable tissue is removed in order to promote healing. The method of debridement depends on the wound, the patient's condition, and the goals of care.

Upon completion of this chapter, the reader will be able to:

1. Identify the methods of wound debridement
2. Choose the appropriate method of debridement for a wound
3. Discuss when debridement is not used for wound care

WHEN IS DEBRIDEMENT OF A WOUND APPROPRIATE?

Wounds are debrided when nonviable tissue is in the wound impeding healing. Such tissues can harbor bacteria and can actually be a barrier to healing. The moist stagnant environment can successfully harbor bacteria—both anaerobic and aerobic—that can then multiply, increasing the bioburden, and lead to infection (Vowden, n.d.). In addition the tissue can mask adequate knowledge about the wound and inhibit contraction and granulation (Leak, 2012).

The methods of debridement include autolytic, bio-surgical, hydro-surgical, mechanical, sharp/conservative sharp, surgical, ultrasonic, and enzymatic. Each method has advantages and disadvantages and the choice depends on the patient and the patient's physician. What is the patient's health status? What does the wound look like? How much debridement is necessary? What are the goals of treatment? Conservative and cost-effective methods are generally chosen before more drastic methods. However, more complex methods may be necessary if the tissue within the wound is not allowing the wound to heal. For some patients this can deter their day-to-day functioning (Leak, 2012).

DEBRIDEMENT METHODS

Autolytic

This method uses the body's own forces to soften and hydrate slough and eschar within the wound. This is accomplished using an occlusive or semi-occlusive dressing. This is a slow process and can leave the wound open to increased bacteria. It is simple, however, and can be done in any setting. The wounds are usually shallow with only a moderate amount of nonvital tissue. This method is a nonselective method of debridement as good tissue can be removed when the dressing is removed.

Bio-Surgical

Larvae (maggots) from the green bottle fly are inserted in the wound to eat dead tissue and bacteria. This method is expensive but it is highly selective as the maggots only ingest the dead tissue and pathogens. Many people do not tolerate this well simply because of the feeling or thought of the larvae.

Hydro-Surgical

A high-powered saline stream is used as a cutting agent. This method selectively and effectively cleans the wound. The procedure and the equipment are highly specialized and require controlled conditions in which personnel are protected from possible contamination from the mist.

Mechanical

Wet to dry saline dressings nonselectively remove eschar and slough when allowed to dry and are removed from the wound. This type of dressing removes good tissue as well, and it requires frequent dressing changes. It is easy and can be done in any setting but it can cause damage to the wound. This method does work and has been used for a long time.

Sharp/Conservative Sharp

This method uses simple surgical tools such as scissors and forceps to remove devitalized tissue from the wound. It can be done at the person's bedside in any setting. It can be done by nurses with specific training from a certified school and if approved by the individual state board of nursing. This method, like surgical debridement, can put the patient at risk and the benefits need to be weighed.

Surgical

Surgical debridement excises the tissue but may take a larger portion where good tissue is removed selectively. The debridement may be done in several steps and is surgery. The patient undergoes pain and is subject to anesthesia. This is accomplished by surgeons, plastic surgeons, or podiatrists. If the wound is causing the patient harm, this surgical method may actually improve the patient status.

Ultrasonic

This method uses an ultrasound probe within the wound or by atomized solution or mist. It is selective, removing only the dead tissue. It is an expensive method and requires a specialized technician or practitioner (Vowden, n.d.).

Enzymatic

Enzymatic debridement uses collagenase, which is the primary enzymatic debriding agent available (papain urea has been used in the past). This type of debridement has been utilized to significantly soften slough and necrotic tissue in the wound. It is conservative and generally can be used on all patients unless they are sensitive to it. The enzyme is placed in the wound essentially "nickel" thick. It is often topped with a dry dressing or moist saline dressing. The dead tissue is removed over time. It is somewhat expensive but less expensive treatments can be used once the dead tissue is removed (Payne, 2008). It can be used on thick eschar but the eschar may need to be opened to allow penetration and therefore may not be the best method.

═══════════════════════════════════*FAST FACTS in a NUTSHELL*

Assess a patient carefully post-debridement. Debridement may cause pain or discomfort. Ensure the site is protected and the patient has sufficient pain medication,

No matter what type of debridement is chosen, it is important to use a multidisciplinary approach to care for the wound. Patients also need to be included in their care. The method depends on their needs and what is best for the wound.

PHOTOGRAPHY—TO SHOOT OR NOT TO SHOOT? THAT IS THE QUESTION

Recent developments in electronic medical records and digital photography have made wound photography seem like the best thing for wound assessment. However, this means of wound documentation is more than just taking a picture of a wound. It also means privacy concerns, patient consent, storage, documentation, and what to do with the photo once taken.

The photo is not a substitute for assessment and documentation but is an enhancement. There are many different opinions regarding the use of photography in wound care and the evidence varies (Wound Ostomy and Continence Nurses Society, 2012). Photography has clear uses in outpatient arenas and plastic surgery clinics to document wound progress. It also can be a good method of documentation in home care as this is a more controlled environment—one nurse to one patient.

In long-term and acute care facilities the evidence is inconclusive. In a hospital that used photography, the method was very ineffective. Nurses took a picture of every mark on a patient's body—all abrasions, moles, skin tears, incontinent dermatitis, and any blemish. There were photos all over, most not making it to the patient's chart. What was the benefit? The hospital had a very high pressure ulcer rate. The photos were not used for anything other than documenting present on admission. They did properly obtain consent but it was a concern because of the amount of photos that were not used appropriately. Not only was there a concern for the patient, but also for the cost and the amount of work for the wound ostomy continence nurse, as the photos should have been reviewed.

This section of this book discussed the methods of treatment for pressure ulcers. Choices vary depending on the patient and what the goal of care is. Using basic methods can be just as effective as the most elaborate and costly form of treatment.

The next section will discuss the quality methods in pressure ulcer assessment and care. Methods to create an atmosphere of patient safety within a facility or agency will be outlined.

Establishing the Environment
of Skin Care Safety

12

Creating an Environment of Skin Safety Throughout the Health Care Facility

In health care facilities or agencies that seek to develop a culture of safety, everyone must be actively involved. Each member of the organization not only reports safety concerns but becomes part of the solution. Everyone knows what is required and applies pressure to those that are not doing the right thing (Institute for Health-care Improvement [IHI], 2011). Whatever the focus, every person becomes involved to resolve a problem or issue. Pressure ulcers are just one piece of the puzzle but when principles of patient safety are resolved, there is a trickle-down effect—other health care issues follow suit.

Upon completion of this chapter, the reader will be able to:

1. Identify two methods to create a culture of safety
2. Discuss what is meant by prevalence and incidence
3. Discuss how nurse rounding can affect the quality of care

METHODS FOR CREATING A SAFE ENVIRONMENT IN PRESSURE ULCER CARE

As part of the culture of safety related to pressure ulcers, prevention methods have been discussed. A pressure ulcer prevention program consists of several proven methods: proper identification of ulcers, assessing risk for development, using pressure ulcer prevention modalities, completing appropriate skin assessment on a regular basis, clear documentation, and appropriately caring for pressure ulcers that do occur so that they heal or do not get worse. The main issue with program development is having everyone do the same thing at all times without variance.

The first method of improving or developing a skin care program is to *hire the right people*. Nurses who have a background not only in skin and wound care but also in managing nursing care would be ideal choices to develop and sustain the program. At least one nurse with this type of knowledge base is needed for success.

Establishing a successful patient care program is *multidisciplinary*. Include all staff members who provide care for the patient. Create a team to look at current findings and what is working and what is not. Frontline staff is the most important part of this team. They know what is being done, what changes are possible, and what will require additional work.

═══════════════════════════*FAST FACTS in a NUTSHELL*

Frontline staff in all types of facilities should be enlisted in program development. They know what works in their daily care routines and then become engaged in the change process.

Next *follow the evidence* in pressure ulcer prevention and skin care. Even though some members may feel certain activities may not work, look at the evidence related to them. There are things that will not work in all facilities but no idea should be shot down; instead, be sure to discuss each suggestion or idea. Put everything on the table. Include the team in current data and practice issues and together identify what changes are needed. Transparency up front will make the problem real. Be sure to discuss why is it a problem, not simply that there is a problem (Dziedzic, 2011).

Include those responsible for budget and economics of the facility in the team process. In this way ideas and plans can be made to achieve results while making appropriate financial decisions. In addition, make sure *all administrators are on board* with the need for change. If they do not walk the talk, the program will not be successful. Ensure that they are active in the change process, not just know about it (IHI, 2011).

Make changes rhythmically but *do not do everything at once.* Follow the evidence within the facility to determine what is a priority. For example, if documentation of present on admission is a major problem, facilitate change in this area first. Do not wait until this is fully established before starting on another piece but continue to work on it as additional changes are instituted.

Have frontline staff *evaluate patient care equipment.* Assess mattresses, lifts, chair cushions, dressings, and treatments. Have staff become active in choosing what will be used on the patients. Educate everyone who will be using the equipment. Have a plan to purchase even if it may not occur immediately. Identify when it can be purchased. Remember, it is for the patient. If something is identified as unsafe or not working it needs to be replaced.

Ensure that all patients have a complete *skin assessment within 8 hours* of entering a facility or agency. Make this a hard stop; the assessment must be complete before anything can be done for the patient except emergent care. Use clear concise documentation tools to make sure this is done. Facilities that use advanced technology and electronic health records have been very successful in this area (Dineen, 2012).

Identify and *agree on a risk assessment tool*. Staff should understand why risk assessment is so important. It has been established that the Centers for Medicare and Medicaid Services (CMS) does require a valid tool for pressure ulcer prevention and that it is utilized on a consistent basis (CMS, 2012). Include this as part of the skin assessment. Use a *visual cue* that identifies patients that are at risk in the institution. Everyone should know about this cue; publicize it.

Make identifying pressure ulcers that are present on admission everyone's responsibility. Everyone needs to understand the importance. Discuss this, review new admissions carefully, and have everyone on board. Talk about this constantly and include it in all patient care conferences (Agency for Healthcare Research and Quality [AHRQ], 2010).

Once the change is made do not assume that it is being carried out. Assess what is being done constantly. If not being done, do education on the spot. Include managers in education and what is occurring. If something is not being done, ensure that all know about it.

If a pressure ulcer does occur, *look at what happened*. Use a team approach to look at the care received by the patient. This is not done in a punitive approach but via education. Humans will make mistakes; humans are not perfect just as the human body is not perfect. In this atmosphere of education, errors in the care of pressure ulcers are monitored, reviewed, and used to make changes (American Nurses Association Board of Directors, 2010).

When processes for change are identified and complete, *look at the next step*. Pressure ulcer prevention can be looked at as a puzzle that is never complete. There is always something that comes up with the human body. For example, a new piece of equipment caused a pressure ulcer. No one knew this would occur but it should not happen again.

BENEFITS OF A SKIN CARE TEAM

Development

A skin care team within an agency or institution is a network of nurses that ensures skin care prevention protocols (bundles) are being carried out in the individual nursing areas. These nurses on the skin care team have the responsibility for enforcing the established protocols. A regular meeting schedule is established for the team to keep up the momentum. Nurses are responsible to attend—it is mandatory and nurse managers must schedule accordingly.

Skin care teams are an excellent method to promote staff education and empowerment. Members from each area are brought together to discuss practice, develop improvement activities, and in general create a network of safety within the facility or agency. The group can be activated to collect and analyze data, educate other staff members about new equipment, and review pressure ulcer occurrences on the individual nursing areas (Dziedzic, 2011).

Nurse Empowerment

These teams can be part of a nursing council network. Established councils have specific responsibilities. Nurses as part of these councils have responsibility for their own practice. They establish patient care protocols and policies. They oversee their own working environment. These councils provide the nurses with empowerment, leadership, growth, vision, and meaningfulness of work. The nurses are part of improvement methods.

It has been established that nursing councils improve quality of care. Nurses are responsible for the care provided and the environment in which it is provided. This improves job satisfaction. Administrators need to support the councils and the decisions of the nurses. Without support the councils will not be sustained (Brody, 2012).

PREVALENCE AND INCIDENCE STUDIES: THE IMPORTANCE OF DATA COLLECTION

Pressure ulcer prevention strategies and establishing a skin care program will improve patient safety, satisfaction, and care. Improvement strategies will yield positive outcomes for patients. It is important, however, to monitor that improvement. It is only through monitoring and data collection that true improvement is noted.

The prevalence of hospital-acquired pressure ulcers varies depending on the agency. In general the benchmark of 0.5 pressure ulcers per 1,000 patient days has been established by the Institute for Healthcare Improvement (IHI, 2011). Many institutions will seek a 0% pressure ulcer goal even though it may not be reasonable. Skin is an organ and organs fail.

When establishing a skin care program it is important to document success. Identify what the pressure ulcer rate was before establishing prevention strategies and what is it after. Use valid data and obtain data from reliable sources. Start small, perhaps establishing prevention methods on one individual unit, but look at it as just a stepping stone and continue improvement efforts.

Established methods for data collection may include prevalence studies. *Prevalence* studies are essentially a snapshot of pressure ulcers in a facility during a given time period. Patients are assessed on a specific day on a regular basis. The skin care team can be part of this project. Both patients who come into the facility and those who acquire pressure ulcers in the facility are included in the study. The number is compared to a national benchmark

Incidence, on the other hand, is the number of hospital acquired pressure ulcers over a period of time. To keep the momentum of pressure ulcer prevention, this is usually done on a monthly basis. These data are reported and analyzed in the facility and as part of the team ("Pressure Ulcer Prevention," 2010).

There are other means to assess progress of the pressure ulcer prevention program. These include discharge audits, discharge skin assessments, and review of assessment and prevention documentation. However, it really is important to collect data in real time. This ensures problems are discussed as they occur ("Pressure Ulcer Prevention," 2010).

THE IMPORTANCE OF NURSE ROUNDING TO PATIENT SAFETY

One evidence-based method to increase patient safety is through *nurse rounding*. Regular and consistent nurse rounding has been proven to decrease patient incidents including falls and pressure ulcers while improving nurse and patient satisfaction. Nurse rounding is purposeful with specific aims in mind. All levels of the nursing unit are involved. Rounds are done at least hourly and "out loud." Staff members who participate state they are doing rounding so the patients know what is occurring.

Each staff person rounds to focus on patient needs. Sometimes rounding is set up so that the nurse rounds during one time period and the nursing assistant in the next (odd versus even hours, for example). Patients are toileted, provided comfort, and repositioned. Patients are told about rounding, care is announced as it is being done. Before rounds are completed patients are asked if they need anything else and are reminded about what time the next rounds will be done. White boards in patient rooms can remind patients about rounding and when to expect the next encounter. In this manner patients' needs are met, their pain is managed, and they are truly positioned frequently. In addition unnecessary call bell use is decreased resulting in improved staff satisfaction (AHRQ Innovations Exchange, 2009).

Once again, patient rounding is a procedure whereby a nursing team member—nurse, caregiver, nursing assistant—rounds on patients on a routine schedule. The usual rounding schedule is every hour to two hours at night. A typical round might include assessing the patient's pain level and administering medicine as needed or alerting an RN. Assistance should also be offered to those who need it to reach the bathroom—actually offer to assist patients to the bathroom on a regular basis to prevent falls and incontinence. The staff member also ensures that the patient is positioned comfortably to prevent pressure ulcers, and places items such as the telephone and call button within the patient's reach. The process helps the staff members become proactive in anticipating patients' needs and fulfilling them before they ask.

Excessive call bell use can cause many problems. Nurses are distracted providing for unsafe care and may actually ignore call bells because they become desensitized to them. Effective nurse rounding decreases call bell use as the patients know when to expect the nurse again. The nurses not only tell the patient when they will return, they document it either on a tablet or white board in the patient's room. The rounds are usually logged, which helps with accountability issues.

It is clear there are many avenues that can be taken not only to prevent skin issues but to facilitate overall patient safety. Through careful nursing intervention at all levels patients can receive the best care possible. The total patient is addressed and although preventing pressure ulcers is just one aspect, the focus on the best possible care will drift into other aspects and the patient will be safe and well cared for.

CONCLUSION

Pressure ulcers can be devastating to patients and costly for the facility. The CMS has changed its method of payment and will not pay for the care of Stage III or Stage IV pressure ulcers if they occur in a facility. It therefore behooves nurses to be aware of what pressure ulcers are and how they occur.

Prevention is multidisciplinary involving all who care for the patient. It starts with identifying those patients who are at risk for pressure ulcer development. This is done on a regular basis along with a thorough skin assessment.

There are many tools used in prevention. Most involve protection of skin, basic skin care, and close observation of pressure points. Nurses use these tools in all settings and facilities need to provide the best care possible with the best equipment possible.

If a pressure ulcer does occur, careful selection of treatment is also necessary to promote healing. This too involves the entire team. Everyone needs to be aware of the protocols and must follow them carefully.

Finally, establishing a network of nurses within the facility or agency goes a long way in pressure ulcer prevention. This team can educate about protocols, new treatment, and equipment. The team also can be part of the data collection that shows the change as a skin care program is developed. It is through these methods that pressure ulcers can be prevented.

Creating a culture of patient safety in a facility or agency requires work and involvement. No one is exempt from prevention practices and change efforts. Change in practice must occur to achieve desired results.

Insanity: doing the same thing over and over again and expecting different results. —Attributed to Albert Einstein, U.S. (German-born) physicist (1879–1955)

Appendices

Elder Abuse Hotlines

Each state has an elder abuse hot line if elder abuse is suspected. If it is an emergency, dial 911 or the local police.

Information and referral is also available from the national Eldercare Locator, a public service of the U.S. Administration on Aging. Call toll-free **1-800-677-1116**. This number is available from Monday through Friday 9 AM-8 PM (except U.S. federal holidays).

State	Report Elder Abuse: Domestic/Community	Report Elder Abuse: Nursing Home/Long-Term Care Facility
Alabama	• 1-800-458-7214	• 1-800-458-7214
	More Information Alabama Adult Protective Services	**More Information** Alabama Department of Senior Services
Alaska	• 1-800-478-9996 (Toll free in Alaska) • Outside of Alaska: 907-269-3666	• 1-800-730-6393 (Toll free in Alaska) • Outside of Alaska: 907-334-4483
	More Information Alaska Adult Protective Services	

(continued)

State	Report Elder Abuse: Domestic/Community	Report Elder Abuse: Nursing Home/Long-Term Care Facility
Arizona	• 1-SOS-ADULT or 1-877-767-2385 • 602-674-4200 • TDD: 1-877-815-8390 **More Information** Arizona Adult Protective Services	• 1-SOS-ADULT or 1-877-767-2385 • 602-674-4200 • TDD: 1-877-815-8390
Arkansas	• 1-800-332-4443 (Toll free in Arkansas) • Outside of Arkansas: 1-800-482-8049 • E-mail: Carolyn. singleton@arkanas.gov • Arkansas Domestic Violence/ Battered Women Hotline: 1-800-332-4443 **More Information** Arkansas Adult Protective Services	• 1-800-582-4887 • In Pulaski County: 501-682-8425 • Fax: 501-682-1967, Attention Complaint Unit • E-mail: complaints .OLTC@arkansas.gov **More Information** • Arkansas Office of Long Term Care, Complaints Unit • Arkansas Long Term Care Ombudsman
California	• 1-888-436-3600 (Toll free in California) • Outside of California: Call County Adult Protective Services **More Information** California Adult Protective Services	• 1-800-231-4024 **More Information** California Long Term Care Ombudsman
Colorado	• 1-800-773-1366	• 1-800-773-1366 or 1-800-886-7689, Ext. 2800 • (303) 692-2800 • E-mail: health.facilities@ state.co.us • Fax: (303) 753-6214 **More Information** Colorado Department of Public Health Nursing Home Complaints Program

(*continued*)

State	Report Elder Abuse: Domestic/Community	Report Elder Abuse: Nursing Home/Long-Term Care Facility
Connecticut	• 1-888-385-4225 or 1-860-424-5241 • After Hours/ Emergency: 2-1-1 (In-State only) • E-mail: lynn.noyes@ po.state.ct.us **More Information** Connecticut Protective Services for the Elderly	• 1-860-424-5241
Delaware	• 1-800-223-9074 **More Information** Delaware Adult Protective Services	• 1-800-223-9074
District of Columbia	• 202-541-3950 **More Information** DC Adult Protective Services	• 202-434-2140
Florida	• 1-800-96-ABUSE or 1-800-962-2873 • TDD/TTY: 1-800-453-5145 • Fax: 1-800-914-0004 **More Information** • Florida Adult Protective Services • Florida Mandatory Reporter Fax Transmittal Form	• 1-800-96ABUSE or 1-800-962-2873
Georgia	• 1-888-774-0152 • 404-657-5250 (Metro-Atlanta) **More Information** Georgia Adult Protective Services	• 1-800-878-6442 • 404-657-5728 (Metro-Atlanta) **More Information** Georgia Office of Regulatory Services

(continued)

State	Report Elder Abuse: Domestic/Community	Report Elder Abuse: Nursing Home/Long-Term Care Facility
Guam	• 671-475-0268 • After Hours: 671-646-4455 (evenings, weekends, holidays)	• 671-475-0268 • After Hours: 671-646-4455 (evenings, weekends, holidays)
Hawaii	• 808-832-5115 (Oahu) • 808-243-5151 (Maui, Molokai, and Lanai) • 808-241-3432 (Kauai) • 808-933-8820 (East Hawaii) • 808-327-6280 (West Hawaii) **More Information** Hawaii Executive Office on Aging	• 808-832-5115 (Oahu) • 808-243-5151 (Maui, Molokai, and Lanai) • 808-241-3432 (Kauai) • 808-933-8820 (East Hawaii) • 808-327-6280 (West Hawaii) **More Information** Hawaii Long-Term Care Ombudsman 808-586-0100
Idaho	• 1-877-471-2777 **More Information** Idaho Adult Protection	• 1-877-471-2777
Illinois	• 1-800-252-8966 (Toll free in Illinois—Voice & TTY) • Outside of Illinois: 217-524-6911 or 1-800-677-1116 (Eldercare Locator) • After Hours Hotline: 1-800-279-0400 • E-mail: ilsenior@aging.state.il **More Information** • Illinois Protective Services for Seniors • Illinois Local Elder Abuse Provider Agency Directory	• 1-800-252-4343 (Toll free in Illinois) • TTY: 1-800-547-0466 • Outside of Illinois: 217-785-0321 **More Information** Illinois Department on Aging

(continued)

State	Report Elder Abuse: Domestic/Community	Report Elder Abuse: Nursing Home/Long-Term Care Facility
Indiana	• 1-800-992-6978 (Toll free in Indiana) • Outside of Indiana: 1-800-545-7763, Ext. 20135 **More Information** Indiana Adult Protective Services	• 1-800-992-6978 (Toll free in Indiana) • Outside of Indiana: 1-800-545-7763, Ext. 20135
Iowa	• 1-800-362-2178 **More Information** Iowa Department of Human Services	• 1-877-686-0027 **More Information** • Iowa Long-Term Care Ombudsman • Iowa Department of Inspections and Appeals, Health Facilities Division
Kansas	• 1-800-922-5330 (Toll free in Kansas) • Outside of Kansas: 785-296-0044 **More Information** Kansas Adult Protective Services	• 1-800-842-0078 • 1-877-662-8362 (Toll free in Kansas) • Outside of Kansas: 785-296-3017 **More Information** Kansas Office of the State Long Term Care Ombudsman
Kentucky	• Elder Abuse Hotline: 1-800-752-6200 • Spouse Abuse Hotline: 1-800-544-2022 **More Information** • Kentucky Cabinet for Health and Family Services • Kentucky Adult Protective Services	• Elder Abuse Hotline: 1-800-752-6200 • Long-Term Care Ombudsman: 1-800-372-2991 • TTY (for hearing impaired): 1-800-627-4702 • Attorney General's Patient Abuse Tip Line: 1-877-ABUSE TIP (1-877-228-7384)

(continued)

State	Report Elder Abuse: Domestic/Community	Report Elder Abuse: Nursing Home/Long-Term Care Facility
		More Information • Office of the Attorney General Medicaid Fraud & Abuse Control Division • Kentucky Office of Inspector General
Louisiana	• 1-800-259-4990 (Toll free in Louisiana) • Outside of Louisiana: 225-342-9722 Adults with Disabilities (Ages 18–59) • 1-800-898-4910 **More Information** Louisiana Elderly Protective Services	• 1-800-259-4990 (Toll free in Louisiana) • Outside of Louisiana: 225-342-9722 Adults With Disabilities (Ages 18–59) • 1-800-898-4910
Maine	• 1-800-624-8404 (Toll free in Maine) • Outside of Maine: 207-532-5047 or 207-287-6083 (After Hours) • TTY: 1-800-624-8404 • TTY After Hours (In-State) 1-800-963-9490 • TTY After Hours (Out-of-State) 207-287-3492 **More Information** Maine Bureau of Elder and Adult Services	• 1-800-383-2441 (Toll free in Maine) • Local/Out-of-State TTY: 207-287-9312 **More Information** Maine Department of Health and Human Services
Maryland	• 1-800-917-7383 (Toll free in Maryland) • Outside of Maryland: 1-800-677-1116 (Eldercare Locator) **More Information** Maryland Adult Protective Services	• 1-800-917-7383 (Toll free in Maryland) • 1-800-AGE-DIAL, Ext. 1091 (Toll free in Maryland) • Outside of Maryland: 410-767-1091 **More Information** Maryland Long Term Care Ombudsman/Elder Abuse Prevention

(continued)

State	Report Elder Abuse: Domestic/Community	Report Elder Abuse: Nursing Home/Long-Term Care Facility
Massachusetts	• 1-800-922-2275 (Toll free in Massachusetts - Voice/TTY) • Outside of Massachusetts: 1-800-AGE-INFO (1-800-243-4636) • TDD/TTY: 1-800-872-0166 **More Information** Massachusetts Elder Protection Services and Programs	• 1-800-462-5540 • 1-800-AGE-INFO (1-800-243-4636) • Massachusetts Attorney General's Elder Hotline: 1-888-AG-ELDER (1-888-243-5337) • TTY: 617-727-0434
Michigan	• 1-800-996-6228 **More Information** Michigan Adult Protective Services	• 1-800-882-6006 **More Information** Michigan Bureau of Health Systems
Minnesota	• 1-800-333-2433 • TDD/TYY: 1-800-627-3529 **More Information** Minnesota Aging Protective Services Unit	• 1-800-333-2433 • TDD/TYY: 1-800-627-3529
Mississippi	• 1-800-222-8000 (Toll free in Mississippi) • Outside of Mississippi: (601) 359-4991 • E-Mail: webspinner@ mdhs.state.ms.us **More Information** Mississippi Adult Protective Services	• 1-800-227-7308 • 1-800-222-8000 (Toll free in Mississippi) • Outside of Mississippi: (601) 359-4991
Missouri	• 1-800-392-0210 **More Information** Missouri Adult Protective Services	• 1-800-392-0210

(continued)

State	Report Elder Abuse: Domestic/Community	Report Elder Abuse: Nursing Home/Long-Term Care Facility
Montana	• 1-800-551-3191 (Toll free in Montana) • Outside of Montana: 406-444-4077 **More Information** Montana Adult Protective Services	• 1-800-551-3191 (Toll free in Montana) • Outside of Montana: 406-444-4077 **More Information** Montana Senior & Long Term Care Division Ombudsman
Nebraska	• 1-800-652-1999 (Toll free in Nebraska) • Outside of Nebraska: 402-595-1324 **More Information** Nebraska Adult Protective Services	• 1-800-652-1999 (Toll free in Nebraska) • Outside of Nebraska: 402-595-1324
Nevada	• 1-800-992-5757 (Toll free in Nevada) • Outside of Nevada: Carson City area: 775-687-4210 • Reno area: 775-688-2964 • Elko area: 775-738-1966 • Las Vegas area: 702-486-3545 **More Information** Nevada Elder Protective Services	• 1-800-992-5757 (Toll free in Nevada) • Outside of Nevada: Carson City area: 775-687-4210 • Reno area: 775-688-2964 • Elko area: 775-738-1966 • Las Vegas area: 702-486-3545
New Hampshire	• 1-800-351-1888 or 603-271-4680 • After Hours: 911 or local police after hours, weekends, or holidays **More Information** New Hampshire Adult Protection Program	• 1-800-442-5640 or 603-271-4375 **More Information** New Hampshire Office of the Long Term Care Ombudsman

(*continued*)

State	Report Elder Abuse: Domestic/Community	Report Elder Abuse: Nursing Home/Long-Term Care Facility
New Jersey	• 1-800-792-8820 (Toll free in New Jersey) • Outside of New Jersey: 609-341-5567 **More Information** New Jersey Adult Protective Services	• 1-800-792-8820 (Toll free in New Jersey) • Outside of New Jersey: 609-341-5567
New Mexico	• 1-800-797-3260 or 505-841-6100 (In Albuquerque)	• 1-800-797-3260 or 505-841-6100 (In Albuquerque)
New York	• 1-800-342-3009 (Toll free in New York) - Press Option 6 **More Information** New York Protective Services for Adults	Nursing Home Complaints • 1-888-201-4563 • E-Mail: nhintake@health.state.ny.us Adult Care Home Complaints • 866-893-6772 **More Information** New York State Department of Health Nursing Homes Adult Care Facilities
North Carolina	• 1-800-662-7030 **More Information** North Carolina Adult Protective Services	1-800-662-7030
North Dakota	• 1-800-451-8693 **More Information** North Dakota Vulnerable Adult Protective Services	• 1-800-451-8693
Ohio	• 866-635-3748 (Toll free in Ohio) • Outside of Ohio: 1-800-677-1116 (Eldercare Locator) **More Information** Ohio Adult Protective Services	• 1-800-342-0533 • TDD: 614-752-6490 • Fax: 614-728-9169 • E-mail: HCComplaints@gw.odh.state.oh.us **More Information** Ohio Department of Health

(continued)

State	Report Elder Abuse: Domestic/Community	Report Elder Abuse: Nursing Home/Long-Term Care Facility
Oklahoma	• 1-800-522-3511 **More Information** Oklahoma Adult Protective Services	• 1-800-522-3511
Oregon	• 1-800-232-3020 • TTY/Voice: 503-945-5811 **More Information** Oregon Adult Protective Services	• 1-800-522-2602 or 503-378-6533 Aging/Developmental Disabilities • 1-800-866-406-4287 or • 503-945-9495 **More Information** • Oregon Long Term Care Ombudsman • Oregon Department of Human Services Office of Investigations
Pennsylvania	• 1-800-490-8505 **More Information** Pennsylvania Protective Services for Adults	• 1-800-254-5164 **More Information** Pennsylvania Department of Health
Puerto Rico	• 787-725-9788 or 787-721-8225	
Rhode Island	• 401-462-0550 • Fax: 401-462-0545 **More Information** Rhode Island Department of Elderly Affairs Protective Services Unit	• 401-785-3340 • Fax: 401-785-3391
South Carolina	• 803-898-7318 **More Information** South Carolina Adult Protective Services	• 803-898-2850

(continued)

State	Report Elder Abuse: Domestic/Community	Report Elder Abuse: Nursing Home/Long-Term Care Facility

South Dakota	• 605-773-3656
	
	More Information
	• South Dakota Adult
	  Protective Services
	• Online Referral/Request
	• South Dakota local adult
	  protection offices
		• 605-773-3656

Tennessee	• 1-888-APS-TENN or
	  1-888-277-8366
	• Knoxville:
	  (865) 594-5685
	• Chattanooga:
	  (423) 634-6624
	• Nashville:
	  (615) 532-3492
	• Memphis:
	  (901) 320-7220
	
	More Information
	Tennessee Adult
	Protective Services
		• 1-888-APS-TENN or
		  1-888-277-8366

Texas	1-800-252-5400
	(Toll free in Texas)
	More Information
	• Texas Adult Protective
	  Services
	• Online Abuse/Neglect/
	  Exploitation Reporting
	  Form
		1-800-458-9858
		(Toll free in Texas)
		Outside of Texas:
		512-834-3784

Utah	• 1-800-371-7897
	  (Toll free in Utah)
	• Outside of Utah:
	  801-264-7669
	• E-mail: vruesch@utah
	  .gov
	
	More Information
	Utah Adult Protective
	Services
		• 1-800-371-7897
		  (Toll free in Utah)
		• Outside of Utah:
		  801-264-7669
		• E-mail: vruesch@utah
		  .gov

(continued)

State	Report Elder Abuse: Domestic/Community	Report Elder Abuse: Nursing Home/Long-Term Care Facility
Vermont	• 1-800-564-1612 • 802-241-2345 • Fax: 802-241-2358 **More Information** • Vermont Adult Protective Services • APS Online Report Form	• 1-800-564-1612 • 802-241-2345 • Fax: 802-241-2358 **More Information** • APS Online Report Form • Vermont Department of Aging & Independent Living
Virginia	• 1-888-83-ADULT or 1-888-832-3858 • Richmond Area: 804-371-0896 **More Information** Virginia Adult Protective Services	• 1-888-83-ADULT or 1-888-832-3858 • Richmond Area: 804-371-0896
Washington	• 1-866-EndHarm or 1-866-363-4276 **More Information** • Washington Aging and Disability Services Administration • Adult Protective Services (APS) Regional Reporting Numbers	• 1-800-562-6078
West Virginia	• 1-800-352-6513 **More Information** West Virginia Adult Protective Services	• 1-800-352-6513
Wisconsin	• 608-266-2536 • E-mail: StopAbuse@dhfs.state.wi.us **More Information** • Wisconsin Department of Health and Human Services • Wisconsin County Elder Abuse Agencies & Help Lines	• 1-800-815-0015 (Toll free in Wisconsin) • Outside of Wisconsin: 608-246-7013 **More Information** Wisconsin Long Term Care Ombudsman
Wyoming	• 1-800-457-3659 (Toll free in Wyoming) • Outside of Wyoming: 307-777-3602	

11

Support Surfaces Available and Manufacturers

Surface	Advantages	Disadvantages	Manufacturers: Type
Air mattress/ overlay	Low maintenance Inexpensive Patient can use in home or in facility Low tech and easy to use Single-patient use, patient can take with them	Need method to inflate Can be punctured Proper inflation must be ensured to prevent bottoming out Can add additional height to the mattress and become a fall risk	*EHOB:* Waffle mattress *Blue Chip:* Stat Air mattress overlay *Drive Medical:* Static Guard air mattress overlay *Invacare:* Air mattress overlay *Stryker:* Soft Care overlay
Gel mattress/ overlay	Low maintenance Resists puncture Easy to clean and can be used on multisurfaces including OR table or ER stretcher Durable	Can be heavy to transport It is important to ensure gel is effective Need to check manufacturer for life of product Can be expensive Little documented research regarding its effectiveness	*Invacare:* Gel mattress overlay *Drive Medical:* Gel mattress overlay *Medline:* Gel mattress overlay *Sierra:* Gel mattress overlay

(*continued*)

Surface	Advantages	Disadvantages	Manufacturers: Type
Foam mattress/ overlay	Light weight No puncturing Can tear No maintenance Single-patient use and can be used in any environment	Holds moisture and heat Fragile; use is limited Cannot clean May retain odors/ bacteria	*Invacare:* Foam mattress overlay *Devon:* Foam mattress pad *Sierra:* Foam mattress overlay *Lumex:* Gold care foam *Geo-Matt-Atlas:* Bariatric foam mattress
Water mattress/bed/ overlay	Common material Easy to clean Can be cooling; however, it does require heating unit	Requires heating unit Heavy Cannot transfer patient easily High maintenance	Water mattress overlay: *Invacare* *Drive Medical* *Blue Chip Medical*
Dynamic overlays	Easy to clean Controls moisture and microclimate Deflates to ease transfers Pump is reusable Patient can use in any setting	Can be punctured Produces noise Power source necessary Higher tech as needs some assembly Can add height to current mattress causing fall risk	*Hill-Rom:* Hill-Rom 300 alternating pressure low air loss *ArjoHuntleigh (KCI):* First step alternating pressure low air overlay; First step low air loss overlay *Invacare:* Low air loss mattress overlay *Stryker:* Low air loss replacement mattress *RoHO:* Low air loss replacement

(continued)

Surface	Advantages	Disadvantages	Manufacturers: Type
Replacement pressure-relieving mattress	Used for all patients No decision tree Staff time reduced Easy to clean Low maintenance Mattresses now reduce friction and shear as well as control moisture	High cost initially It is important to replace per manufacturers' recommendation as they may lose effectiveness Higher cost mattress may be necessary to include moisture control and reduce friction and shear	*Hill-Rom:* Accu-Max replacement pressure-relieving mattress *ArjoHuntleigh:* Atmos Air 3000 mattress replacement system *Stryker:* Pioneer stretcher pad replacement pressure relief technology *Medline:* Equalizer therapeutic mattress
Low air loss bed	Controls allow for assistance with positioning; head and feet can be elevated Reduces friction and shear Controls moisture May have cooling effect	Requires electricity source May be difficult to use in home Expensive and requires set up Often rented, creating extra steps for staff It may be difficult to assist patient out of bed, even deflated Patient must be assisted to position Noisy	*ArjoHuntleigh (KCI):* Kin Air Med Surge *Hillrom:* Versicare 500 therapeutic surface

(continued)

Surface	Advantages	Disadvantages	Manufacturers: Type
Air fluidized bed	Lowest interface pressure, relieves pressure consistently Reduces friction and shear Reduces moisture	Heavy Because of the moisture balance, can actually cause dehydration or fluid and electrolyte imbalance Warm climate Difficult to transfer and help patient out of bed, decreasing mobility	*Hill-Rom:* Clinitron Air Fluidized Therapy Bed; Rite-Hite Clinitron Air Fluidized Therapy

Source: Agency for Healthcare Research and Quality, 2010; Dorner, 2009; Salcido & Lorenzo, 2012.

Chair Surfaces Available and Manufacturers

Chair cushions come in a variety of materials, many of them the same as support surface. Consider a chair cushion for most patients, especially if they are out of bed in the chair for a period of time. Outpatients are also vulnerable to skin breakdown.

Cushion Type	Manufacturer
Air	EHOB
	Medline
	ROHO
	Stryker
Gel foam	ROHO
	Invacare
	New York Orthopedic
	Hermell
	Medline
Mattress quality	ArjoHuntleigh (KCI)
	Posey

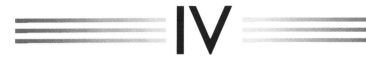

IV

Choosing the Appropriate Dressing

Choosing the appropriate dressing depends on the assessment of the wound and the characteristics of the wound bed. A moist environment promotes cell proliferation and allows epithelial cells to migrate. The type of dressing depends on the goal of healing.

Dressing	Advantages	Disadvantages	Company–Dressing
Gauze: • Draining wounds • Protection of delicate or surgical wounds • Packing due to space in the wound • Packing of wound to assist with debridement • Wounds with tunneling or undermining to fill space	• Inexpensive • Easily obtainable • Many different forms • Can be used easily with topical products • Absorbent	• Needs to be secured • Frequent dressing changes often necessary causing trauma or frequent intervention • Not used alone to maintain moist wound bed	*Smith & Nephew:* Conformant wound veil PROFORE wound contact layers *Covidien:* Curity *BSN Medical:* Cutisorb Ultra Super-Absorbent dressing *Mölnlycke:* Mepore *Holister:* Restore *ConvaTec:* Surpress absorbent padding
Transparent film: • Clear two sided sheet • Protects wound • Visualize wound • Creates seal preventing microbes from entering wound • Most often used for superficial wounds and burns • Use as secondary dressing	• Protect wound or area from friction • Clear film allows to see wound • Many Sizes • Flexible • Seals wound • Infrequent dressing changes—5 to 7 days	• May stick to some wounds and delicate skin • Adhesive may be difficult to remove • No absorption • No oxygen for wound • Not for draining wounds or moist burns	*3M Health Care:* 3M Tegaderm *Systagenix:* BIOCLUSIVE select transparent film dressing *Hartman USA:* Hydrofilm transparent film dressing *Mölnlycke Health Care:* Mepore film *Smith & Nephew:* OPSITE *ReliaMed:* ReliaMed film dressing

(continued)

Dressing	Advantages	Disadvantages	Company–Dressing
Foam: • Used for high draining wounds • Highly absorbent • Does not stick to wound • Can be used for protection • Protection under compression wraps • Can be used for deep cavity wounds and large pressure ulcers • Use for wounds with tunnels, undermining	• Large amount of sizes and shapes • Can be obtained in large dressing sizes • Easy to apply and remove • Provides comfort • Very absorbent, decreasing frequency of dressing changes	• May become too absorbent and dry wound bed • Not used with non-draining wounds except for protection • Often needs a secondary dressing • Needs to be assessed and changed at least every 3 to 5 days to avoid damage to surrounding skin or wound	*3M Health Care:* 3M Tegaderm *Smith & Nephew:* Allevyn *ConvaTec:* Aquacel foam dressing; Versiva XC Gelling foam dressings *Coloplast:* Biatin *Covidien:* Kendall Ultra-Soft foam dressings *Mölnlycke:* LYOFOAM; Mepilex Border Sacrum Self-Adherent foam dressing *Hartman USA:* Permafoam foam dressing *Ferris:* PolyMem; PolyMem Max Wound Care Dressings; PolyMem Wic Wound Cavity fillers: Shapes by PolyMem *ReliaMed:* ReliaMed foam dressing *Holister Wound care LLC:* Restore *Derma Sciences Inc.:* XTRASORB foam dressings

(continued)

Dressing	Advantages	Disadvantages	Company–Dressing
Composite dressing: • Dressing made of different products often with increased results • Many have a surrounding nonadherent or semi-adherent border • Maintains moist wound environment • Large ulcers and wounds including leg ulcers (semi-adherent may not be appropriate for this use) • Can be used for chronic, open or superficial wounds	• Comfort • Prevents friction • Maintains and promotes moist environment of wound • Protects wound from microbes • Comfort in application and removal	• Some may dry wound • Peri-wound skin may become too moist • Can cause trauma with removal • Use on intact skin	*3M Health Care:* 3M Meidpore+Pad Soft Cloth Adhesive Wound Dressings *Mölnlycke Health Care:* Alldress; Mesalt *ConvaTec:* AQUACEL; CombiDerm *Covidien:* Curity Sodium Chloride Dressings *ReliaMed:* ReliaMed Composite Barrier Dressings *MPM Medical Inc.:* Repel Waterproof Composite Wound Dressing
Hydrocolloid: • Used for low or moderate draining wounds • Can be used under compression wraps • Used to pad bony prominence • Can be used for necrotic wounds promoting debridement • Can be used for all pressure ulcers	• Many sizes and shapes • Absorbs moderate amount of drainage • Easy to apply • Provides comfort • Can provide insulation and protection	• Can stick to wound or surrounding skin • Needs to be removed carefully to prevent trauma • Drainage under dressing can be odorous misleading caregiver to think wound is infected	*3M Health Care:* 3M Tegaderm *Coloplast:* Comfeel *ConvaTec:* DuoDERM *Covidien:* Kendall Alginate Hydrocolloid dressing; Kendall Hydrogel Impregnated Gauze; Kendall Hydrogel wound dressings

Dressing	Advantages	Disadvantages	Company–Dressing
			Derma Sciences: MEDIHONEY Honeycolloid dressing *Systagenix:* NU-DERM Hydrocolloid wound dressing *ReliaMed:* ReliaMed Hydrocolloid wound dressing *Smith & Nephew:* Replicare *Hollister Wound Care LLC:* Restore
Hydrogel: • Used for wounds with no or minimal drainage • Provides moisture to dry wounds • Used for all ulcers in wound bed to promote moist environment • Keeps grafts, burns, donor sites moist • Can be used for necrotic wounds with some debriding properties • Allows oxygen and water vapor into wound	• Rehydrates wounds promoting cell growth • May be soothing • Provides comfort reducing friction • Removes easily and by cleansing wound • Comes in variety of forms including gels and sheets	• Not for very moist wounds • Minimal absorption • Usually requires secondary dressing • Most often daily dressing changes	*HARTMAN USA:* AquaClear Gel Sheet dressing *Southwest Technologies Inc.:* Comfort-Aid; Elasto-Gel; Horseshoe-shaped dressings *Derma Sciences:* Dermagran *MPM Medical Inc.:* Excel Gel Hydrogel dressing *Smith & Nephew:* Intrasite Gel Amorphous Hydrogel dressings *ReliaMed:* ReliaMed Hydrogel Sheet dressings

(continued)

Dressing	Advantages	Disadvantages	Company–Dressing
			Hollister Wound: Care LLC: Restore Hydrogel dressing *Spenco:* Spenco 2nd Skin AquaHeal *Medline:* Tenderwet *Coloplast:* Triad Hydrophillic Dressings
Alginate: • Made of soft fibers that are not woven • Dressing absorbs drainage and turns to gel • Can have additives such as calcium or antimicrobial silver • Used for moderate to high absorption • Can pack wound with dressing • Can be used for draining ulcers	• Absorbs large amount of drainage • Removes easily not sticking to wound • Amount of dressing changes are decreased	• Can dry wounds with minimal drainage • Requires secondary dressing • Removed with wound cleansing, may be uncomfortable	*Coloplast:* SeaSorb Soft AG Alginate *UDL Labs:* Sorbsan *Derma Science Inc.:* Algicell *ConvaTec:* KALTOSTAT Calcium Sodium Alginate *Hartman:* Sorbalgon Calcium Alginate *ReliaMed:* Cal Alginate CMC dressings *Covidien:* Kendall Health CareCurasorb *3M Tegaderm:* High Integrity Alginate *Systagenix:* Nu-Derm Alginate *Deroyal:* Deroyal Alginate

Dressing	Advantages	Disadvantages	Company–Dressing
			Mölnlycke Health Care: Melgisorb *Smith & Nephew:* Algisite *Medline Industries:* Maxorb *Hollister:* Restore Calcium Alginate dressing
Collagen: • Promotes healing • Absorbs drainage (amount depends on dressing) • Can be used for chronic wounds promoting environment for cell growth • Can be used for ulcers and large wounds • Dressings provide protection	• Maintains moist environment • Promotes fibroblast cells • Protects from external environment	• Often not the least expensive choice • Requires secondary drainage • Application may be difficult requiring specific manufacturer's instructions	*Hartman:* Collasorb *Human Biosciences:* Skin Temp II dressing sheets *Covalon Technologies:* ColActive Plus Collagen *Systagenix:* Fibracol Plus Collagen wound dressing; Promogram Prisma *Medline Industries:* Purcol Plus AG Collagen Dressing *MPM Medical:* Triple Helix Collagen Dressing *Smith & Nephew:* Biostep Collagen matrix *Coloplast:* Woun'dres Collagen Hydrogel

(continued)

165

Dressing	Advantages	Disadvantages	Company–Dressing
Hydrofiber: • Dressing turns into gel with drainage like alginate • Highly absorbent • Promotes a healthy wound environment • Can be packed into wounds and used on dry wounds when moistened with normal saline	• Often most cost effective for large exudate wounds • Comfortable conforming to shape of wound/body • Decreased frequency of dressing changes	• Not for use with petroleum products • Sensitivity may occur if patient is sensitive to silver	*ConvaTec:* AQACEL hydrofiber; Versiva XC nonadhesive gelling foam
Antimicrobial: • Various forms of dressing such as gel, film, foam or composite impregnated with antimicrobial solution. • Used for infected wounds • Can be used initially on surgical sites • Can be used with burns or superficial wounds	• Reduces infection risk • Used with topical medicine • Can be layered for comfort • Can reduce infection • Promotes comfort by reducing infection	• Use secondary dressing • Often frequent dressing changes • Not used with people with iodine sensitivity	*Systagenix:* Johnson & Johnson Biopatch Antimicrobial dressing *Mölnlycke:* Mepilex soft silicone absorbent dressing *Covidien Kendall Health Care:* AMD Antimicrobial Island Dressing; AMD Antimicrobial Foam dressing; Telfa AMD non-adhering antimicrobial dressing *Vomaris:* Procellera Antimicrobial dressing *Smith & Nephew:* Acticoat 7 Day Antimicrobial Barrier wound dressing

(continued)

Dressing	Advantages	Disadvantages	Company–Dressing
Silver dressings: • Dressings with silver that prevent or kill microbes • Available in many forms and can be used for *Staph* infections • Can be used under compression or other dressings • Also used for wounds that are prone to infection	• Reduces infection • Are often cost-effective alternative • Promote comfort through reducing infection	• Often need secondary dressing • May need frequent dressing changes • May need moisture to activate silver component • Not for use with patients that have silver sensitivity	*MediPurpose:* MediPurpose MediPlus Super foam AG *Derma Sciences Inc.:* Algicel AG Antimicrobial Sliver Dressing *Covalon Technologies:* ColActive Plus silver collagen dressing *Deroyal:* Algidex AG Silver alginate wound dressing *Mölnlycke:* Mepilex Border AG antimicrobial dressing *Hartman:* Sorbalgon AG dressing *Smith & Nephew:* Allevyn AG antimicrobial border dressing *3M Health Care:* Alginate AG silver dressing *ConvaTec:* Aquacel AG Hydrofiber dressing *Coloplast:* SeaSorb Ag Alginate BiatinAg Adhesive Foam antimicrobial dressing

Source: Baranoski, 2012; Bergquist-Beringer, 2011; EPUAP and NPUAP, 2009.

V

E-Resources

Resources for pressure ulcer identification, treatment, and prevention:

Identification and prevention:

1. www.npuap.org/resources
2. www.ihi.org/offerings/MembershipsNetworks/ MentorHospitalRegistry/Pages/PressureUlcerPrevention .aspx
3. www.guideline.gov/content.aspx?id=24492
4. www.mayoclinic.com/health/bedsores/DS00570/ DSECTION=prevention
5. www.health.nsw.gov.au/resources/quality/pdf/pres sure_ulcers_commcare.pdf
6. www.cms.gov/Medicare/Medicare-Fee-for-Service-Payment/HospitalAcqCond/index.html?redirect=/ hospitalacqcond
7. search.ahrq.gov/search?q=pressure+ulcers&entqr= 0&output=xml_no_dtd&proxystylesheet=AHRQ_ GOV&client=AHRQ_GOV&site=default_ collection&x=0&y=0

Treatment:

1. www.woundsinternational.com/journal/issue/1/
   practice-development
2. www.nice.org.uk/nicemedia/pdf/CG029publicinfo
   .pdf
3. www.hopkinsmedicine.org/gec/series/wound_care
   .html
4. cms.hhs.gov/medicare-coverage-database/details/
   technology-assessments-details.aspx

References

Agency for Healthcare Research and Quality. (2008). Preventing pressure ulcers and skin tears. *Evidence-based geriatric nursing protocols for best practice* guideline. Retrieved December 2, 2012, from guideline.gov/content.aspx?id=12262

Agency for Healthcare Research and Quality. Innovations Exchange. (2009). *Hourly rounds help reduce falls, pressure ulcers, call light use and contribute to rise in patient satisfaction.* Springfield, IL: Memorial Health System. Retrieved December 1, 2012, from www.innovations.ahrq.gov/content.aspx?id=3204

Agency for Healthcare Research and Quality. (2010, March 30). *Pressure ulcers.* Retrieved from AHA health care exchange http://www.guideline.gov/content.aspx?id=36059

Agency for Healthcare Research and Quality. (n.d.). *Preventing pressure ulcers in hospitals: A toolkit for improving quality care.* Retrieved December 12, 2012, from www.ahrq.gov/research/ltc/pressureulcertoolkit/putool3.htm

American Nurses Association Board of Directors. (2010, January 28). *Position Statement: Just culture.* Retrieved January 3, 2013, from nursingworld.org/psjustculture.

Antokal, S. B., et al. (2012, November 20). *Friction induced skin injuries—Are they pressure ulcers?* A National Pressure Ulcer Advisory Panel (NPUAP) White Paper, 1–3.

Arnold-Lolng, B. S. (2010, February). The use of Dakin's solution in chronic wounds: A clinical perspective case series. *Journal of Wound Ostomy and Continence Nursing, 37*(1), 94–104.

Ayello, E. (2012, July). *ConsultGeriRN.org.* Retrieved June 5, 2013, from Nursing Standard of Practice Protocol: Pressure Ulcer Prevention and Skin Tear Prevention: consultgerirn.org/topics/pressure_ulcers_and_skin_tears/want_to_know_more

Baranoski, S. (2012, February). Wound dressings an evolving art and science. *25.* Retrieved January 2, 2013, from www.nursingcenter.com/pdf.asp?AID=1293384

Barker, L. G. (2011, February). Hospital malnutrition: Prevalence, identification and impact on patients and the health care system. *International Journal of Environmental Research and Public Health, 8,* 514–527.

Bergquist-Beringer, S. (2011). Outcome and assessment information set data that predict presure ulcer development in older adult home health patients. *Advances in Skin and Wound Care, 24*(6), 404–414.

Black, J. E. (2011, February). Pressure ulcers: Avoidable or unavoidable? Results of the National Pressure Ulcer Advisory Panel Consensus Conference. *Ostomy Wound Management.* Retrieved December 1, 2012, from www.o-wm.com

Braden, B. (1998). *The Braden Scale for Predicting Pressure Ulcer Risk.* Retrieved November 3, 2013, from www.bradenscale.com

Brienza, D. K. (2010). A randomized clinical trial on preventing pressure ulcers with wheelchair cushions. *Journal of the American Geriatrics Society, 58*(12), 2308–2314.

Broderick, N. (2009, October). Understanding chronic wound healing. *The Nurse Practitioner, 34*(10) 17–22.

Brody, A. B. (2012, January). Evidence based nursing councils: Potential path to staff empowerment and leadership growth. *Journal of Nursing Administration, 42*(1), 28–33.

Cafardi, S., & Centers for Medicare & Medicaid Services. (2012, April). *Examination of the accuracy of coding pressure ulcers.* (p. 1–18).

Centers for Medicare & Medicaid Services. *www.CMS.com.*

Centers for Medicare & Medicaid Services. (2012, August 27). *Medicare policy regarding pressure reducing support surfaces.* Retrieved June 5, 2013, from Medicare Learning Network:www.cms.gov/

Outreach-and-Education/Medicare-Learning-Network-MLN/
MLNMattersArticles/downloads/SE1014.pdf

Centers for Medicare & Medicaid Services. (2012, September 7). Retrieved June 1, 2013, from Present on Admission (POA) by Acute Inpatient Prospective Payment System (IPPS) Hospital: www.cms.gov/Medicare/Medicare-Fee-for-Service-Payment/HospitalAcqCond/index.html?redirect=/HospitalAcqCond/

ConvatecUSA. (2012). *Stages of a pressure ulcer.* Retrieved from www.convatec.com/en/cvtus-stagespuus/cvt-cntsngcol/0/detail/10138/1464/1547/stages-of-a-pressure-ulcer.html

DeMarco, S. (n.d.). *Wound and pressure ulcer management.* Johns Hopkins Medicine. Retrieved November 27, 2012, from www.hopkinsmedicine.org/se/util/display_MODULE

DermNet NZ. (2012). N. Z. Incorporated, Producer). Retrieved January 1, 2012, from www.dermnetnz.org/dermatitis/intertrigo.html

Dineen, J. (2012, February 28). Health reforms by the numbers. *Strategy+Business.* Retrieved January 3, 2013, from www.strategy-business.com/article/12101?gko=95c10

Dorner, B. P. (2009). *The role of nutrition in pressure ulcer prevention and treatment: National Pressure Ulcer Advisory Panel (NPUAP) white paper.* NPUAP.

Drolet, A. D. (2012, September 13). Move to improve the feasibility of using an early mobility protocol to increase ambulation in the intensive and intermediate care settings. *Journal of the American Physical Therapy Association.* Retrieved November 30, 2012, from ptjournal.apta.org/content/early/2012/09/11/ptj.20110400.abstract

Dziedzic, M. (2011, September 30). Preventing pressure ulcers in the acute care setting. *Mosby's Nursing Consult.* doi:www.nursingconsult.com/nursing/clinical-updates/full-text?clinical_update_id=209547

European Pressure Ulcer Advisory Panel (EPUAP) and National Pressure Ulcer Advisory Panel (NPUAP). (2009). *Prevention and treatment of pressure uclers: Quick reference guide.* Washington, DC: National Pressure Ulcer Advisory Panel.

Foster, M. (2013). *Wound Care Principles and Products.* Retrieved June 1, 2013, from www.apsna.org/--wound-care

Goodwin, C. K. (2011, July-Aug). Anatomy and Physiology of the skin. *Journal of the Dermatology Nurses' Association, 3*(4), 203–213.

Gray, M. B.-E. (2011, May/June). Moisture associated skin damage overview and pathophysiology. *Journal of WOCN, 38*(3), 233–241.

Healthcare Cost and Utilization Project. (2011, August). *An example of using present on admission data: CMS-defined hospital acquired conditions in all-payer data.* Retrieved June 1, 2013, from www.hcup-us.ahrq/gov/datainnovations/clinicaldata/ExampleofUsing POA-CMSHACsuingall-payerdata.jsp

He, W., Liu, P., & Chen, H. L. (2012). The Braden Scale cannot be used for assessing pressure ulcer risk in surgical patients: A meta analysis. *Ostomy Wound Management, 58*(2), 34–40.

Hess, C. (2008). Performing a skin assessment. *Advances in Skin and Wound Care, 21*(8), 392.

Hess, C. (2009, January). Taking steps to prevent pressure ulcers. *Nursing 2013, 39*(1), 61.

Hurd, T. (n.d.). *Nutrition and wound care: Management and prevention.* Retrieved June 3, 2013, from Wound Care Canada: cawc.net/images/upload

Institute for Healthcare Improvement. (2011). *Pressure ulcer prevention.* Retrieved January 3, 2013, from www.ihi.org/offerings/membershipsnetworks/mentorhospitalregistry/pages/pressureulcerprevention.aspx

Institute for Healthcare Improvement. (2011, August 18). *Relieve the pressure and reduce harm.* Retrieved from www.ihi.org/knowledge/Pages/ImprovementStories/RelievethePressureandReduce Harm.aspx

Institute for Health Care Improvement. (2011). *Creating a culture of safety.* Retrieved January 3, 2013, from www.ihi.org/knowledge/Pages/Changes/DevelopaCultureofSafety.aspx

Katz, M. (2012). *Wound care.* Retrieved January 2, 2013, from www.nursingceu.com/courses/395/index_nceu.html

King, L. (2012, September/October). Developing a progressive mobility activity program. *Orthopedic Nursing, 31*(5), 253–262.

Kottner, J., & Dassen, T. (2010, June). Pressure ulcer risk assessment in critical care: Interrater reliability and validity of the Braden and Waterflow scales and subjective ratings in two intensive care units. *International Journal of Nursing Studies, 47*(6), 671–677.

Lab studies on line. (2013). Retrieved from labtestsonline.org

Leak, K. (2012, February 22). *Ten top tips for wound debridement.* Retrieved January 2, 2013, from http://www.woundsinternational.com/

practice-development/how-to-ten-top-tips-for-wound-debridement.

Little, M. (2013). Nutrition and skin ulcers. *Clinical Nutrition, 16*(1), 136.

Lyder, C. (2008). Pressure ulcers: A patient safety issue. In R. Hughes (Ed.). Agency for Healthcare Research and Quality. Retrieved December 28, 2012, from www.ncbi.nih.gov/books/NBK2650/?report=printable

Mayo Clinic. (2012). *Hyperbaric oxygen therapy.* Retrieved January 2, 2013, from www.mayoclinic.com/health/hyperbaric-oxygen-therapy/MY00829/DSECTION=risks

Middlesex Hospital's community e-newsletter. (2011, July). The NICHE program: Improving the care of elderly patients. Retrieved June 1, 2013, from middlesexhospital.org/newsletter/evita/july2011/niche.html

Muir, M. (2009). *Essentials of a bariatric handling program.* Retrieved June 1, 2011, from www.nursingworld.org/MainMenuCategories/ANAMarketplace/ANAPeriodicals/OJIN/TableofContents/Vol142009/No1Jan09/Bariatric-Patient-Handling-Program-_1.aspx

National Pressure Ulcer Advisory Panel. (2009). *Pressure ulcer staging revised.* Retrieved April 25, 2008, from www.npuap.org

The Norton Pressure Score: Risk-assessment scoring system. (1962). Retrieved from www.nutrition411.com/wrc/pdf/w0513_norton_presure_sore_risk_assessment_scale_scoring_system.pdf

Nurse Leader Insider. (2009, March 2). *Tool of the month: Minimize pressure ulcers by preventing fricion and shear.* Retrieved June 3, 2013, from www.hcpro.com

Occupational Safety and Health Administration. (2009, March). *Guidelines in nursing homes.* Retrieved June 5, 2013, from US Department of Labor: www.osha.gov/ergonomics/guidelines/nursinghome/final_nh_guidelines.html

Pajula, C., & Osborn, E. (2008, January/February). Prevention and early detection of pressure ulcers in hospitalized patients. *Journal of Wound Ostomy & Continence Nursing, 35*(1), 65–75.

Payne, W. S., et al. (2008, April 7). Enzymatic debridement agents are safe in wounds with high bacterial bioburdens and stimulate healing. *Open Access Journal of Plastic Surgery-ePlasty.* Retrieved January 2, 2013, from http://www.ncbi.nlm.nih.gov/pmc/articles/PMC2311452.

Peterson, B. (2011, March/April). *Patient mobilization*. Retrieved from www.psqh.com

Pressure ulcer. (2013). *The New York Times Health Guide*. Retrieved from http://health.nytimes.com/health/guides/injury/pressure-ulcler/overview.html

Pressure ulcer prevention: Prevalence and incidence in context (2010). *A consensus document*. Retrieved January 2, 2013.

Provider Synergis LLC. (2010, February 10). *Anti-fungal topical review*. Retrieved from www.oregon.gov/oha/pharmacy/therapeutics/docs/ps-2010-02-antifungals-topical.pdf

Rush, A. (2009). Bariatric care: Pressure ulcer prevention. *Wound Essentials, 4*, 68–74.

Salcido & Lorenzo, C. T. (2012, January 18). *Pressure ulcers and wound care: Support surfaces and specialty beds*. Retrieved June 3, 2013, from Medscape Reference: emedicine.medscape.com/article/310284-overview

Sibbald, G. K. (2011, December). Pressure ulcer staging revisited: Superficial changes and deep pressure ulcer framework. *Advances in Skin & Wound Care, 24*(32), 571–580.

Skretkowicz, V. (Ed.). (2010). *Florence Nightingale's Notes on Nursing and Notes on Nursing for the Labouring Classes*. New York, NY: Springer Publishing Company.

Swezy, L. (2011, May 5). Preventing heel ulcers: Simple methods and identifying risk factors. *Wound Source*. Retrieved from www.woundsource.com/blog/preventing-heel-pressure-ulcers-simple-methods-and-identifying-risk-factors

United Seating and Mobility. (2012). *Medicare Part B coverage for therapeutic mattresses*. Retrieved from www.unitedseating.com/store/pages/Medicare-Part-B-Coverage-Criteria-for-Therapeutic-Mattresses

University of Texas School of Nursing. (2004). *How to identify and prevent pressure ulcers*. Inservice Education.

Vanderbilt University Medical Center. (2012, April). *Accreditation & standards*. Retrieved June 5, 2013, from Joint Commission Survey Ready: www.mc|.vanderbilt.edu/documents/mysite/files/AccredNewsletter.pdf

Victorian Government Health Information. (2012). *Mobility, vigor and self care*. Retrieved June 9, 2013, from Best Care for Older People Everywhere Toolkit: www.health.vic.gov.au/older/toolkit/

Vieira, E. D. (2008). Safety in bariatric patient transfers. *The Open Critical Care Medicine Journal, 1*, 48–53.

Vowden, K. (n.d.). *Debridement made easy.* Wounds UK. Retrieved January 2, 2013, from www/wounds-uk.com/debridement-made-easy&print

Wake, W. (2010, Summer). Pressure ulcers: What clinicians need to know. *The Permanente Journal, 14*(2), 56–60.

Warner, R. (2009, November 17). *Cool mist humidifiers: The best dry skin treatment.* Retrieved June 3, 2013, from Ezine articles: ezinearticles.com/?Cool-Mist-Humidifiers---The-Best-Dry-Skin-Treatment&id=3285143

Waterlow, J. (2005). The *Waterlow score.* Retrieved November 3, 2013, from http://www.judy-waterlow.co.uk/waterlow_score.htm

Waterlow, J. (2009). *Pressure ulcer causes.* Retrieved from www.judy-waterlow.co.uk/pressure-sore-causes.htm

World Health Organization. (2013). *Controlling the global obesity epidemic.* Retrieved from www.who.int/nutrition/topics/obesity/en/

World Health Organization. (2013). *Ultraviolet Radiatiom and the INTERSUN Program: The Known Health Effects of UV.* Retrieved from www.who.int/uv/faq/uvhealtfac/en/index1.html

Wound Ostomy and Continence Nurses Society. (2010, June). *Guideline fo prevention and management of pressure ulcers.* Mount Laurel, NJ. Retrieved from guideline.gov/content.aspx?id=23868

Wound Ostomy and Continence Nurses Society. (2006–2011). *WOCN Society Position Statement Pressure Ulcer Staging.* Mount Laurel, NJ: Author. Retrieved 2012, from www.wocn.org

Wound Ostomy and Continence Nurses Society. (2009, March 24). *Position paper: Avoidable vs unavoidable pressure ulcers.* Retrieved from c.ymcdn.com/sites/www.wocn.org/resource/resmgr/docs/wocn-avoidable-unavoidable_p.pdf

Wound Ostomy and Continence Nurses Society. (2012). *Photography in wound documentation: Fact sheet.* WOCN wound committee. Retrieved January 2, 2013, from c.ymcdn.com/sites/www.wocn.org/resource/collection/E3050C1A-FBF0-44ED-B28B-C41E24551CCC/Photography_in_Wound_Documentation-Fact_Sheet_(2012).pdf

Wounds International (International Review). (2010). *Pressure ulcer prevention: Pressure, shear, friction and microclimate in contect.* London: Wound International Enterprise House.

Index

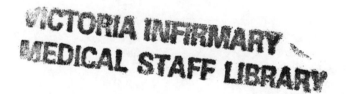